Articular Cartilage

Editor

ERIC C. McCARTY

CLINICS IN
SPORTS MEDICINE

www.sportsmed.theclinics.com

Consulting Editor
MARK D. MILLER

July 2017 • Volume 36 • Number 3

ELSEVIER

1600 John F. Kennedy Boulevard • Suite 1800 • Philadelphia, Pennsylvania, 19103-2899

http://www.theclinics.com

CLINICS IN SPORTS MEDICINE Volume 36, Number 3
July 2017 ISSN 0278-5919, ISBN-13: 978-0-323-53154-2

Editor: Lauren Boyle
Developmental Editor: Donald Mumford

Clinics in Sports Medicine (ISSN 0278-5919) is published quarterly by Elsevier Inc., 360 Park Avenue South, New York, NY 10010-1710. Months of issue are January, April, July, and October. Business and Editorial Offices: 1600 John F. Kennedy Blvd., Ste. 1800, Philadelphia, PA 19103-2899. Customer Service Office: 3251 Riverport Lane, Maryland Heights, MO 63043. Periodicals postage paid at New York, NY and additional mailing offices. Subscription prices are $343.00 per year (US individuals), $627.00 per year (US institutions), $100.00 per year (US students), $389.00 per year (Canadian individuals), $774.00 per year (Canadian institutions), $235.00 (Canadian students), $475.00 per year (foreign individuals), $774.00 per year (foreign institutions), and $235.00 per year (foreign students). Foreign air speed delivery is included in all *Clinics* subscription prices. All prices are subject to change without notice. **POSTMASTER:** Send address changes to *Clinics in Sports Medicine*, Elsevier Health Sciences Division, Subscription Customer Service, 3251 Riverport Lane, Maryland Heights, MO 63043. Customer Service (orders, claims, online, change of address): Elsevier Health Sciences Division, Subscription Customer Service, 3251 Riverport Lane, Maryland Heights, MO 63043. **Tel: 1-800-654-2452 (U.S. and Canada); 314-447-8871 (outside U.S. and Canada). Fax: 314-447-8029. E-mail: journalscustomerservice-usa@elsevier.com (for print support); journalsonlinesupport-usa@ elsevier.com (for online support).**

Reprints. For copies of 100 or more of articles in this publication, please contact the Commercial Reprints Department, Elsevier Inc., 360 Park Avenue South, New York, NY 10010-1710. Tel.: 212-633-3874; Fax: 212-633-3820; E-mail: reprints@elsevier.com.

Clinics in Sports Medicine is covered in *MEDLINE/PubMed (Index Medicus) Current Contents/Clinical Medicine, Excerpta Medica,* and *ISI/Biomed.*

Contributors

CONSULTING EDITOR

MARK D. MILLER, MD
S. Ward Casscells Professor, Head, Division of Sports Medicine, Department of
Orthopaedic Surgery, University of Virginia, Charlottesville, Virginia; Team Physician,
James Madison University, Director, Miller Review Course, Harrisonburg, Virginia

EDITOR

ERIC C. McCARTY, MD
Chief of Sports Medicine and Shoulder Surgery, Associate Professor, Department of
Orthopedics, University of Colorado School of Medicine, Director of Sports Medicine,
Head Team Physician, University of Colorado Athletics Department, Adjunct
Associate Professor, Department of Integrative Physiology, University of Colorado,
Boulder, Colorado; Head Orthopedic Team Physician, University of Denver Athletics
Department, Denver, Colorado

AUTHORS

JAY C. ALBRIGHT, MD
Surgical Director of Sports Medicine, Assistant Professor, Department of Orthopedics,
Children's Hospital Colorado, University of Colorado, Aurora, Colorado

KATHRYN L. BAUER, MD
Orthopedic Surgeon, Children's Health Andrews Institute for Orthopedics and Sports
Medicine, Plano, Texas

CAMILA B. CARBALLO, MSc
Tissue Engineering, Repair, and Regeneration Program, Hospital for Special Surgery,
New York, New York

JORGE CHAHLA, MD
Steadman Philippon Research Institute, Vail, Colorado

BRIAN J. COLE, MD, MBA
Professor, Department of Orthopedic Surgery, Rush University Medical Center, Chicago,
Illinois

CHRISTOPHER M. COLEMAN, MD
Instructor Fellow, Department of Radiology, University of Colorado Hospital, Aurora,
Colorado

ARIEL KIYOMI DAOUD, BA
Department of Orthopedics, Children's Hospital Colorado, University of Colorado, Aurora,
Colorado

JONATHAN A. FLUG, MD, MBA
Assistant Professor, Department of Radiology, University of Colorado Hospital, Aurora, Colorado

TIGRAN GARABEKYAN, MD
Southern California Hip Institute, North Hollywood, California

ANDREAS H. GOMOLL, MD
Cartilage Repair Center, Brigham and Women's Hospital, Chestnut Hill, Massachusetts

BETINA B. HINCKEL, MD, PhD
Missouri Orthopaedic Institute, University of Missouri, Columbia, Missouri

CALE A. JACOBS, PhD, ATC
Research Assistant Professor, Department of Orthopaedic Surgery and Sports Medicine, University of Kentucky, Lexington, Kentucky

MATTHEW J. KRAEUTLER, MD
Department of Orthopedics, University of Colorado School of Medicine, Aurora, Colorado

ROBERT F. LaPRADE, MD, PhD
Steadman Philippon Research Institute, Vail, Colorado

CHRISTIAN LATTERMANN, MD
Vice Chair for Clinical Research, Professor, Department of Orthopaedic Surgery and Sports Medicine, University of Kentucky, Lexington, Kentucky

TIMOTHY LEROUX, MD
Fellow, Orthopedic Sports Medicine, Department of Orthopedic Surgery, Rush University Medical Center, Chicago, Illinois

NANCY MAJOR, MD
Professor, Department of Radiology, University of Colorado Hospital, Aurora, Colorado

ERIC C. MAKHNI, MD, MBA
Division of Sports Medicine, Department of Orthopedic Surgery, Henry Ford Health System, West Bloomfield, Michigan

CHAITU MALEMPATI, DO
Assistant Professor, Department of Orthopaedic Surgery and Sports Medicine, University of Kentucky, Lexington, Kentucky

OMER MEI-DAN, MD
CU Sports Medicine and Performance Center, University of Colorado, Boulder, Colorado

YUSUKE NAKAGAWA, MD, PhD
Tissue Engineering, Repair, and Regeneration Program, Hospital for Special Surgery, New York, New York; Center for Stem Cells and Regenerative Medicine, Tokyo Medical and Dental University, Tokyo, Japan

SHANE J. NHO, MD, MS
Division of Hip Preservation Surgery, Rush University Medical Center, Chicago, Illinois

CLAYTON W. NUELLE, MD
Department of Orthopaedic Surgery, University of Missouri, Columbia, Missouri

CECILIA PASCUAL-GARRIDO, MD
Assistant Professor, Department of Orthopedics, Washington University, St Louis, Colorado

SOURAV K. PODDAR, MD
Director, Primary Care Sports Medicine, Associate Professor, Departments of Family Medicine and Orthopedics, University of Colorado School of Medicine, Aurora, Colorado

JOHN D. POLOUSKY, MD
Surgical Director and Chief of Pediatric Orthopedics, Children's Health Andrews Institute for Orthopedics and Sports Medicine, Plano, Texas

SCOTT A. RODEO, MD
Tissue Engineering, Repair, and Regeneration Program, Hospital for Special Surgery, New York, New York

BRYAN M. SALTZMAN, MD
Resident, Department of Orthopedic Surgery, Rush University Medical Center, Chicago, Illinois

ICHIRO SEKIYA, MD, PhD
Center for Stem Cells and Regenerative Medicine, Tokyo Medical and Dental University, Tokyo, Japan

SETH L. SHERMAN, MD
Assistant Professor, Department of Orthopaedic Surgery and the Missouri Orthopaedic Institute, University of Missouri, Columbia, Missouri

AUSTIN V. STONE, MD, PhD
Department of Orthopedic Surgery, Wake Forest School of Medicine, Winston-Salem, North Carolina

EMIL THYSSEN, BS
School of Medicine, University of Missouri, Columbia, Missouri

GIFT C. UKWUANI, MD
Division of Hip Preservation Surgery, Rush University Medical Center, Chicago, Illinois

ARMANDO F. VIDAL, MD
Associate Professor, Department of Orthopedics, University of Colorado School of Medicine, Aurora, Colorado

LUKE WIDSTROM, DO
Sports Medicine Fellow, Department of Family Medicine, University of Colorado School of Medicine, Aurora, Colorado

FRANK B. WYDRA, MD
Department of Orthopedics, University of Colorado School of Medicine, Aurora, Colorado

PHILIP J. YORK, MD
Department of Orthopedics, University of Colorado School of Medicine, Aurora, Colorado

WILLIAM ZUKE, BS
Division of Hip Preservation Surgery, Rush University Medical Center, Chicago, Illinois

Contents

The most challenging aspects in treating articular cartilage injury include
identifying the cellular and molecular mechanism(s) that lead to matrix
changes and the differentiation and dedifferentiation behavior of chondrocytes, and understanding how they affect the structural integrity of the
articular cartilage and tissue remodeling. Several treatment strategies
have been proposed. A better understanding of the signaling pathways
and growth and transcription factors for genes responsible for chondrogenesis is an important component in the development of new therapies
to prevent cartilage degeneration or promote repair to replicate the physiologic and functional properties of the original cartilage.

MRI remains the optimal imaging modality to evaluate cartilage injuries in
the athlete. As these injuries have no intrinsic healing capacity, early and
accurate noninvasive diagnosis remains integral to determining the most
appropriate treatment option in this class of patients. Although surgical
success depends primarily on clinical outcomes, MRI evaluation can provide pertinent information regarding the status of the surgical repair and
the progression of cartilage disease.

Nonoperative options for articular cartilage injury are pervasive but have
not shown to be curative. Recommendations for low-impact exercise
and weight loss provide benefit and are a foundation for the treatment of
osteoarthritis. Judicious use of NSAIDs and acetaminophen can be appropriate for pain management. Topical NSAIDs may be a treatment option
with fewer side effects than its oral counterpart. Additionally, viscosupplementation injections are useful for mild to moderate knee osteoarthritis,
whereas short-term pain relief is provided by intra-articular corticosteroid
injections. Future studies to individualize treatment options based on patient phenotype and genotype may hold promise.

Biological treatments for articular cartilage repair have gained in popularity in the past decade. Advantages of these therapies include minimal invasiveness, improved healing time, and faster recovery. Biological therapies for cartilage repair include platelet-rich plasma, bone marrow aspirate concentrate, and cell-based therapies. These methods have the added benefit of containing growth factors and/or stem cells that aid in recovery and regeneration. The purpose of this article is to review the current cartilage treatment options and the existing literature on outcomes, complications, and safety profile of these products for use in the knee and hip joints.

Although osteochondritis dissecans (OCD) has been a recognized condition for more than 100 years, our understanding of the etiology, natural history, and treatment remains poorly characterized. OCD most commonly affects the knee, followed by the elbow and ankle. Adolescents and young adults are most commonly affected. Patients present with vague, often intermittent symptoms and generally have no history of acute injury. Although diagnosis can be made with plain radiographs, treatment decisions are generally based on MRI. Skeletal maturity and stability of the OCD lesion determine treatment. Treatments range from immobilization and activity restriction to operative therapies. Clinical indications are discussed.

Osteochondral autologous transplantation (OAT) is a treatment strategy for small and medium sized focal articular cartilage defects in the knee. This article reviews the indications, surgical techniques, outcomes, and limitations of OAT for the management of symptomatic chondral and osteochondral lesions in the knee joint.

Articular cartilage damage remains a significant cause for early osteoarthritis in adolescents and young adults. After chondroplasty alone, the mainstay procedure for cartilage injuries is microfracture. Although in small lesions this may be successful long-term, positive results of treating larger lesions this way are less certain. This inconsistency in outcomes has led to augmentation of these defects with scaffolding for autograft regeneration or for allograft cartilage to fill the defect with a hyaline cartilage. This discussion includes current techniques for the addition of scaffolding to the microfracture defect for larger lesions, the rationale, and preliminary results.

There is an increasing need for articular cartilage restoration procedures. Hyaline cartilage lacks intrinsic healing capacity. Persistent osteochondral defects can lead to early and rapid degenerative changes. Microfracture and autologous chondrocyte implantation provide reasonable outcomes for smaller defects without bone loss. However, these techniques have limited effectiveness for lesions greater than 4 cm^2 or with significant bony involvement. Ostochondral allografts provide an option for these lesions. This article reviews osteochondral allografts for articular defects. Emerging options provide different approaches to difficult cartilage defects. We discuss current screening, procurement, and storage methods, surgical techniques, outcomes, and bacterial/viral transmission.

Focal chondral defects of the knee are common and can significantly impair quality of life. The autologous chondrocyte implantation technique has evolved over the past 20 years; the newest third-generation technique is matrix-induced autologous chondrocyte implantation. Physical examination is important to characterize location and source of pain and identify associated injuries. Imaging studies allow characterization of the lesions, identification of associated lesions, and alignment. Conservative measures should be exhausted before proceeding with surgical treatment. Steps of surgical treatment are diagnostic arthroscopy and biopsy, chondrocyte culture, and chondrocyte implantation. The techniques and their outcomes are discussed in this article.

Isolated, full-thickness chondral lesions of the glenohumeral joint are a significant pathology encountered by laborers, athletes, and the elderly. A thorough history should be obtained in any patient presenting to the office with shoulder pain and concern for the etiology being an articular cartilage defect. The first-line imaging should include plain radiographs of the glenohumeral joint; MRI and CT can be ordered as necessary to provide greater detail. Typically, the initial treatment of glenohumeral chondral disease is nonsurgical; however, many surgical treatment options have been refined to provide pain relief, create reparative tissue, or restore the articular surface.

Patients with articular cartilage lesions of the hip may present with pain and symptoms that may be vague in nature and onset. Therefore, a thorough history and physical examination should be performed for every patient presenting with hip pain and/or disability. The management may be operative or nonoperative. Nonoperative management includes a trial of rest and/or activity modification, along with anti-inflammatory medications, physical therapy, and biologic injections. Operative treatment in the form of arthroscopic techniques continues to decrease morbidity and offer innovative solutions and new applications for microfracture, ACT, and AMIC.

Patients with early osteoarthritis (OA) have been reported to have inferior outcomes with an increased prevalence of early failure after cartilage procedures. The underlying reasons for this failure are likely multifactorial, including a chronic synovial and chondrogenic process, which is confounded by persistent muscle weakness and altered pain processing for those with increased preoperative symptom duration. Pain, radiographic changes, patient-reported outcomes, and macroscopic changes on arthroscopic evaluation or MRI can assist clinicians in identifying the early OA knee to both aid in clinical decision making and create realistic postoperative expectations for patients.

CLINICS IN SPORTS MEDICINE

RELATED INTEREST

Orthopedic Clinics of North America, January 2017 (Vol. 48, Issue 1)
Controversies in Fracture Care
Frederick M. Azar, James H. Calandruccio, Benjamin J. Grear, Benjamin M. Mauck,
Jeffrey R. Sawyer, Patrick C. Toy, and John C. Weinlein, *Editors*
Available at: http://www.orthopedic.theclinics.com/

THE CLINICS ARE AVAILABLE ONLINE!
Access your subscription at:
www.theclinics.com

Foreword
Articular Cartilage

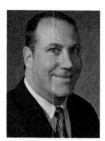

Mark D. Miller, MD
Consulting Editor

"If we consult the standard Chirurgical Writers from Hippocrates down to the present Age, we shall find, that an ulcerated Cartilage is universally allowed to be a very troublesome Disease; that it admits of a Cure with more Difficulty than carious Bone; and that, when destroyed, it is not recovered."[1]

Special thanks to Dr Eric McCarty and his team of articular cartilage experts who have made giant strides in order to attempt to prove Dr Hunter's almost three-century-old characterization wrong. In his Preface, Eric referred to "gray-haired sports medicine physicians." As one of those myself, I certainly have more to learn, especially regarding this troublesome disease.

This issue of *Clinics in Sports Medicine* goes way beyond merely scratching the surface; it is a complete treatise on our current knowledge of articular cartilage diagnosis and treatment. Basic science and imaging are discussed as well as all treatment options, beginning with nonoperative treatment and then includes well-established options (microfracture, autograft, allograft, and cell-based) as well as newer procedures (including biologic options and "microfracture plus"). Although the knee is traditionally

Clin Sports Med 36 (2017) xiii–xiv
http://dx.doi.org/10.1016/j.csm.2017.04.002
0278-5919/17/© 2017 Published by Elsevier Inc.

the target for these procedures, this issue also includes treatment options for the shoulder, hip, elbow, and ankle.

Great job on a troublesome topic—there is still much to learn and much to discover!

Mark D. Miller, MD
Division of Sports Medicine
Department of Orthopaedic Surgery
University of Virginia
400 Ray C. Hunt Drive, Suite 330
Charlottesville, VA 22908-0159, USA

E-mail address:
mdm3p@virginia.edu

REFERENCE

1. Hunter W. On the structure and diseases of articulating cartilages. Trans R Soc Lond 1743;42B:514–21.

Preface

Articular Cartilage: The Search for the Holy Grail of Treatment and Restoration

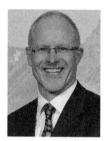

Eric C. McCarty, MD
Editor

It is with great pleasure that I introduce this issue of *Clinics in Sports Medicine* focused on the topic of Articular Cartilage. More than ever the subject of Articular Cartilage is drawing interest in sports medicine physicians, researchers, and the public. It is a hot topic, with the treatment and science constantly evolving as we try to treat a structure that does not heal on its own after injury.

The topic of articular cartilage is an ever-changing one, and the science on articular cartilage is constantly being updated. This issue serves as an excellent update and resource for the current state-of-the-science and treatment options for articular cartilage wear in 2017.

The subject of articular cartilage conjures some type of sentiment for every sports medicine practitioner. Cartilage means something to almost everyone involved in sports medicine, whether as a competitive athlete or recreational sports enthusiast, or a practitioner, or a researcher. Every sports medicine practitioner has had a patient that has been affected by an injury to the articular cartilage, and the term "articular cartilage injury" or "damage" invokes a different image for everyone. There is such a wide spectrum that articular cartilage injury encompasses: from minimal fibrillations of superficial cartilage wear to small cartilage defects to large defects, and finally, to full-blown and widespread grade IV changes of generalized osteoarthritis. Not only have we all had patients that have been affected with a cartilage issue but also many of us have been affected either directly by incurring a cartilage injury or indirectly as a family member has been affected.

As wide as the spectrum of articular cartilage disease is, the treatment of the cartilage lesions might be even wider. The treatment can be challenging as there is a wide continuum of lesions and many options for treatment from injections to arthroplasty with no gold standard for the treatment. In addition, there are so many factors that

Clin Sports Med 36 (2017) xv–xvi
http://dx.doi.org/10.1016/j.csm.2017.04.001
0278-5919/17/© 2017 Published by Elsevier Inc.

sportsmed.theclinics.com

affect the treatment, including but not limited to comorbidities, alignment, stability, biologic factors, patient expectations, activity level, previous surgeries, cost of procedures, and insurance issues.

The interest among the public is at an all-time high. Information on the Internet is expansive, both good and bad. With so much of the public affected, the interest in treatment options, particularly nonsurgical options, has significantly risen and so have the unproven treatments and the public's willingness to pay large amounts of cash in hope of finding the "Holy Grail" treatment. Much is needed in science and studies to understand the nonsurgical options.

A recent concept introduced by Dr Fred Nelson is the idea that a joint should be considered an organ. As one uses this perspective, then any cartilage injury is not treated in isolation. There is a milieu of issues that can contribute to the health of articular cartilage, including mechanical alignment of the joint, stability, and factors that increase the mechanical pressures in the joint (ie, removal of meniscus tissue in the knee). It is beyond the scope of this issue to go into all of the issues associated with the health of the joints and factors that contribute to articular cartilage injury and health, but suffice it to say, this issue of *Clinics in Sports Medicine* will delve into the salient factors involved in the science of articular cartilage, the imaging, the physiology of early osteoarthritis, and the myriad of nonoperative and operative options of articular cartilage restoration for the most affected joints in the body (knee, hip, shoulder).

A big thanks to Mark Miller for allowing me the opportunity to corral and bring together my colleagues and leaders of sports medicine for this issue, and, to my sweet wife, Miriam, who puts up with long hours and often late nights so that the "calling" of the academic mission of efforts such as this can be fulfilled.

I applaud the renowned experts and leaders in the ever-changing field of articular cartilage that have worked hard and made terrific thoughtful contributions to this issue. As you read this issue of *Clinics in Sports Medicine*, enjoy the content, the information, and ideas that have been presented. These articles represent the latest information for the practitioner on the topic of articular cartilage. There is something for everyone: for the new student just trying to understand the concepts to the gray-haired sports medicine physician with many years of experience trying to garner new information. As you read, also understand that this is an evolving subject and that information is constantly being renewed and evaluated. It will be very interesting to see what the *Clinics in Sports Medicine* issue of articular cartilage will look like two decades from now. I would expect that many of the articles will be obsolete, and there will be many more articles on the biological treatment of cartilage disease with an emphasis on disease-modifying modalities. Enjoy this issue. It is my hope that the contents spur thoughts and ideas that will help shape the research and techniques that contribute to the articular cartilage issue of *Clinics in Sports Medicine* in the year 2027.

Many blessings to you as you learn more in these readings and in your pursuit for the Holy Grail in the treatment of articular cartilage injury.

Eric C. McCarty, MD
University of Colorado
CU Sports Medicine
Champions Center
2150 Stadium Drive
Boulder, CO 80309, USA

E-mail address:
Eric.McCarty@ucdenver.edu

Basic Science of Articular Cartilage

Camila B. Carballo, MSc[a], Yusuke Nakagawa, MD, PhD[a,b], Ichiro Sekiya, MD, PhD[b], Scott A. Rodeo, MD[a,*]

KEYWORDS

- Articular cartilage • Chondrocytes • ECM • Chondrogenesis • Cartilage injuries

KEY POINTS

- Articular cartilage has highly organized structure composed of 4 zones. The chondrocyte phenotype, cell shape, and the extracellular matrix (ECM) structure vary among the 4 zones.
- The biomechanical behavior of articular cartilage is viewed as a biphasic medium.
- Chondrocytes are responsible for maintenance of cartilage homeostasis through ECM production.
- The cytokine–matrix metalloproteinase relationship seems to contribute to the intrinsic process of cartilage degeneration.
- Several strategies have been studied to identify the optimal method to maintain the chondrocyte differentiation status and to prevent mesenchymal stem cell hypertrophy and maintain their ECM environment.

BASIC MACROSCOPIC AND MICROSCOPIC STRUCTURE OF HYALINE CARTILAGE

The hyaline cartilage is the most abundant type of cartilage in the body. It is responsible for the bone formation in the embryo (endochondral ossification) and in adults, it can be found in costal cartilages, respiratory system (trachea), and covering the bone articular surface (articular cartilage). A gross inspection of healthy articular cartilage from the joints of a young adult mammal shows the surface to be smooth, shiny, and dense white (**Fig. 1**A). The color of immature articular cartilage is somewhat bluish, and in aged animals, the cartilage becomes yellowish. Articular cartilage has a highly organized structure composed of 4 zones: the superficial (tangential) zone, middle (transitional) zone, deep (radial) zone, and calcified zone (see **Fig. 1**B). The chondrocyte phenotype, cell shape, and the extracellular matrix (ECM) structure

The authors have nothing to disclose.
[a] Tissue Engineering, Repair, and Regeneration Program, Hospital for Special Surgery, 535 East 70th Street, New York, NY 10021, USA; [b] Center for Stem Cells and Regenerative Medicine, Tokyo Medical and Dental University, 1-5-45 Yushima, Bunkyo-Ku 113-8510, Tokyo, Japan
* Corresponding author.
E-mail address: rodeos@hss.edu

sportsmed.theclinics.com

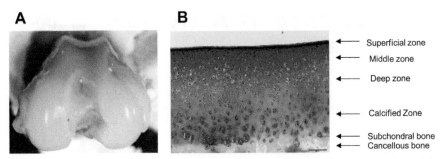

Fig. 1. Normal cartilage of the distal femur in a young adult pig. (*A*) Gross specimen. The surface of the cartilage is dense white, glistening, and smooth. (*B*) Histology stained with safranin-O (original magnification, ×40). Matrix and chondrocytes are well organized in each zone. The superficial zone has no safranin-O staining. In the middle zone, where safranin-O staining appears, the cells are rounded or ovoid and seem to have random distribution; in contrast, in the deep zone, the cells are arranged in short columns.

vary among the different zones.[1,2] The dominant load carrying structural components of the ECM are collagen (75% of the dry weight) and proteoglycan (20%–30% of the dry weight), the concentrations of which vary with depth from the articular surface.[3,4] Collagen content is highest in the superficial zone, decreasing by 20% in the middle and deep zones. Proteoglycan content is lowest at the superficial zone, increasing by as much as 50% into the middle and deep zones.[3,4]

The superficial zone typically stains for fast green only, and does not for safranin-O. Note the lamina splendens, a layer of fine collagen fibers at the very surface of this zone (**Fig. 2**A), in which the cells are elongated and tangentially arranged (**Fig. 2**B). In the middle zone, where safranin-O staining first appears, the cells are rounded or ovoid and seem to have a random distribution, whereas in the deep zone the cells are arranged in short columns[5] (**Fig. 2**C).

The tidemark is a thin basophilic line that usually can be seen in a slide stained with hematoxylin and eosin, represents the boundary between the mineralized and unmineralized regions, and separates the deep zone from the calcified zone.

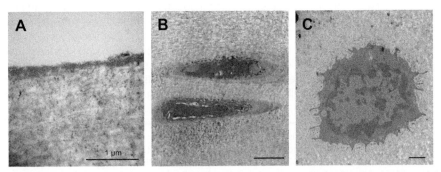

Fig. 2. Transmission electron microscopy images of the distal femur in a normal rat. (*A*) Lamina splendens, the fine fibers and filaments in the surface of articular cartilage. (*B*) Elongated cells in the superficial zone. (*C*) A round cell in the deep zone. (*Reprinted from* Nakagawa Y, Muneta T, Otabe K, et al. Cartilage derived from bone marrow mesenchymal stem cells expresses lubricin in vitro and in vivo. PLoS One 2016;11(2):e0148777; with permission.)

ARTICULAR CARTILAGE FUNCTION

Articular cartilage is a thin layer of specialized connective tissue with unique visco-elastic characteristics. The principal functions are to provide a smooth, lubricated surface for low-friction articulation and to facilitate the transmission of loads to the underlying subchondral bone. The specific material characteristics allow cartilage to carry high contact forces, and to disperse the resulting compressive stresses to the underlying subchondral bone. To keep the shear stresses low, complex lubrication mechanisms are facilitated during articulation. These keep friction and wear low when the joint surfaces glide on each other.

The biomechanical behavior of articular cartilage is best understood when the tissue is viewed as a biphasic medium. Articular cartilage consists of 2 phases: a fluid phase and a solid phase. Water is the principal component of the fluid phase, contributing up to 80% of the wet weight of the articular cartilage. Inorganic ions such as sodium, calcium, chloride, and potassium are also found in this phase. The solid phase is characterized by the ECM, which is porous and permeable.[5,6] The relationship between proteoglycan aggregates and interstitial fluid provides compressive resilience to articular cartilage through negative electrostatic repulsion forces.[7-9] The initial and rapid application of articular contact forces during joint loading causes an immediate increase in interstitial fluid pressure. This local increase in pressure causes the fluid to flow out of the ECM, generating a large frictional drag on the matrix.[5-7,10] When the compressive load is removed, interstitial fluid flows back into the cartilage. The low permeability of articular cartilage prevents fluid from being quickly squeezed out of the matrix.[11] The 2 opposing bones and surrounding cartilage confine the cartilage under the contact surface. These boundaries are designed to restrict mechanical deformation.

Synovial fluid (SF) also plays a pivotal role in the biomechanical behavior, lubrication, and nutrition of the articular cartilage, being the major source of nutrients, because articular cartilage nature is avascular. SF is a dynamic reservoir of proteins derived from cartilage and synovial tissue; thus, its composition may serve as a biomarker that reflects the health and pathophysiologic condition of the joint. The boundary–lubricant ability of SF and the effective boundary friction in cartilage are achieved by the combination of synergistic action of all 3 SF constituents, namely, hyaluronic acid, lubricin (superficial zone protein), and phospholipids at physiologic concentrations.[12,13]

THE MATURE ARTICULAR CARTILAGE EXTRACELLULAR MATRIX

The ECM of mature articular cartilage production is related directly to the chondrocyte volume or function, and is composed of 3 major types of macromolecules: fibers (collagen and elastin), proteoglycans, and glycoproteins, which are synthesized and maintained by chondrocytes.

Collagen is the principal fiber found in the ECM and many different types of collagen molecules are expressed in mature articular cartilage. Collagen II is the predominant collagen type in hyaline cartilage (>90%), but hyaline cartilage also contains collagen III (~10%), collagen IX (1%), collagen XI (3%), collagen VI (<1%, exclusively in the pericellular matrix surrounding chondrocytes), which can play an important role in regulating chondrocyte mechanotransduction, thus mediating the mechanical properties of the pericellular matrix in an age-related manner.[14] Collagen X is found only in the hypertrophic cartilage, in the calcified layer.[15] Associated with these fibrillar components are the noncollagenous elements of the ECM ground substance, including glycosaminoglycans (GAGs), proteoglycans, and glycoproteins. GAGs are carbohydrates made up of repeating disaccharides units, resulting in 6 major subunits in articular cartilage: chondroitin sulfate 4 and 6, keratin sulfate, dermatan sulfate, heparan sulfate, and hyaluronan (or hyaluronic acid). They are negatively charged, repelling each other while attracting ions (eg, Ca^{++} and Na^+) and water,[16,17] ensuring their main functional characteristics of water absorption and maintenance of the mechanical properties and hydration of the ECM.

Proteoglycans are hydrophyllic proteins that have 1 or more GAG chains covalently attached to a protein core. Among the aggregating proteoglycans family, aggrecan is the largest and forms a multimolecular complex with hyaluronan, where GAGS keratin sulfate and chondroitin sulfate are attached and which is stabilized by link proteins.[18] The other member of this family is versican, which is present at much lower levels.

The family of small leucine-rich repeat proteoglycans include biglycan and decorin, which contain dermatan sulfate chains, and fibromodulin and lumican, which contain keratan sulfate chains.[19] Other types of proteoglycans present in mature articular cartilage also include perlecan[20,21] and lubricin (superficial zone protein or PRG-4).[5,22]

Numerous other noncollagenous proteins can be detected in the articular cartilage ECM. They may be divided into 2 subgroups according to their function in the matrix as structural and regulatory proteins.[18] Structural proteins include cartilage oligomeric protein (or thrombospondin-5), thrombospondin-1 and -3, cartilage matrix protein (matrilin-1) and matrilin-3, fibronectin, tenascin-C, and cartilage intermediate layer protein. The regulatory proteins group may influence cell metabolism rather than playing a structural role in the matrix, and this category includes the following proteins: gp-39/YKL-40, matrix Gla protein, chondromodulin-I and -II, cartilage-derived retinoic acid-sensitive protein, and growth factor as transforming growth factor-β (TGF-β) and bone morphogenic proteins.

ARTICULAR CHONDROCYTE BIOLOGY

Chondrocytes are specialized mesenchymal cells that occupy only 2% of the total tissue volume of the articular cartilage.[23] Chondrocytes are responsible for ECM production and maintenance of cartilage homeostasis by producing enzymes, growth factors, and inflammatory mediators. Different signaling pathways, cytokines, and growth and transcription factors regulate chondrocyte function and mediate cartilage and bone formation and homeostasis, chondrocyte differentiation during skeletal development (**Fig. 3**), and maintenance of mature articular cartilage health in adults.[24,25] Any injury or degenerative process that disturbs this homeostatic balance may result in release of the chondrocyte from growth arrest and their activation with aberrant expression of proinflammatory and catabolic genes.[26]

INFLAMMATORY MEDIATORS

The ability of chondrocytes to degrade ECM constituents depends on their capacity to synthesize and secrete proteinases. Under physiologic conditions, the controlled activity of these enzymes is required for proper tissue remodeling. Among the proteinases responsible for cleavage of collagen and proteoglycans are matrix metalloproteinases (MMPs) and disintegrin-metalloproteinases with thrombospondin motifs (ADAMTS), respectively and to a lesser extent, other types of enzymes such as elastase and cathepsin.

Degeneration of articular cartilage and development of osteoarthritis (OA) leads to mechanical and inflammatory stresses that activate common signal transduction pathways in all joint tissues. Proinflammatory cytokines such as interleukin-1 beta (IL-1β) and tumor necrosis factor-alpha induce the expression of prostaglandins, nitric

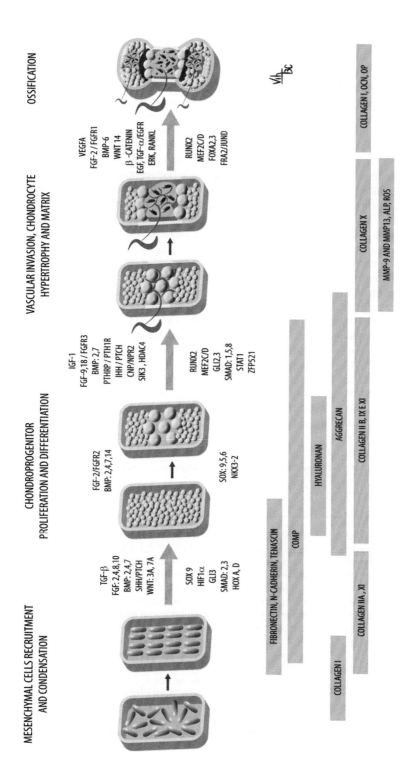

oxide, cyclooxygenase, and MMPs[27] and may also induce other proinflammatory cytokines, such as IL-6, IL-8,[28,29] IL-17, and IL-18.[25,30]

TGF-β plays a crucial role in embryonic cartilage development through its role in the chondrogenic transformation of primitive mesenchymal condensations, and TGF-β also affects mature articular cartilage as a homeostasis regulator for both subchondral bone and articular cartilage. Recently, it has been demonstrated that altered TGF-β signaling, with high concentrations of TGF-β1, is involved in the pathogenesis of OA development, whereas inhibition of TGF-β1 attenuates cartilage degeneration in mice.[31] Handorf and colleagues[32] also showed that TGF-β1 was capable of inducing Ihh expression in chondrocyte cultures derived from human bone marrow stromal cells. These data suggest that TGF-β1 plays a role in both cartilage health and disease.

Of the 26 MMPs identified, MMP-13 has the highest expression of any proteinase in OA and can degrade both collagen II and aggrecan. Other collagenases including MMP-1 and MMP-14 are important mediators in the OA process. Stromelysin (MMP-3) and gelatinases (MMP-2 and MMP-9) have also been reported to play a role in collagen degradation. In addition, the aggrecanases ADAMTS-4 and ADAMTS-5 seem to be the primary mediators of aggrecan cleavage.[33,34] All of these aforementioned proteinases, mainly MMP-13, seem to be emerging as important therapeutic targets in OA, and some studies have been done in an attempt to identify potential therapeutic strategies. A novel regulatory pathway involving the transcriptional regulator CITED2 may contribute to MMP regulation in chondrocytes under moderate levels of flow-induced shear, because the upregulation of CITED2 coincided with downregulated expression of MMP-1 and MMP-13 in human C28/I2 chondrocytes.[35] Furthermore, E74-like factor 3 was identified as a procatabolic factor that may contribute to cartilage remodeling and degradation by regulating MMP-13 gene transcription[36] and IKKa/CHUK has shown the ability to drive articular chondrocyte differentiation by acting as a positive effector of MMP-13 via 2 mechanism involving the upregulation of MMP-10 (stromelysin-2) messenger RNA and the suppression of tissue inhibitor of metalloproteinase-3 accumulation.[37] Wang and colleagues[38] recently demonstrated that alpha 2 macroglobulin, a serum protease inhibitor that seems to be a master inhibitor of many types of cartilage-degrading enzymes, acts not only by

---

Fig. 3. Scheme of chondrogenesis during long bone development (endochondral ossification). The sequence of different stages shows the growth factors, differentiation factors, and some of their receptors above the arrows. Underneath each arrow, the relevant transcription factors involved are listed, and the extracellular matrix proteins expressed at each step of this process are highlighted in orange. ALP, alkaline phosphatase; BMP, bone morphogenetic protein; CNP, C-type natriuretic peptide; COMP, cartilage oligomeric matrix protein; EGF, epidermal growth factor; ERK, extracellular signal-regulated kinase; FGF, fibroblast growth factor; FGFR, fibroblast growth factor receptor; FOXA, forkhead box A; FRA2, (FOS)-related antigen 2; HDAC4, histone deacetylase 4; HIF1a, hypoxia-inducible transcription factor 1 alpha; HOX, homeobox transcription factor; IGF, insulin-like growth factor; IHH, Indian hedgehog; MEF2, myosin enhancer factor 2; MMP, matrix metalloproteinase; NKX3-2, NK3 homeobox 2; NPR2, natriuretic peptide receptor; OCN, osteocalcin; OP, osteopontin; PTCH, patched; PTHrP, parathyroid-hormone related protein; RANKL, RANK-Ligand; ROS, reactive oxygen species; Runx2, runt-related transcription factor 2; SHH, sonic hedgehog; SIK3, salt-inducible kinase 3; SOX9, sex-determining region Y-type high-mobility group box 9; STAT, signal transducer and activator of transcription 1; TGF, transforming growth factor; VEGFA, vascular endothelial growth factor A; Wnt, *Drosophila* segment polarity gene wingless and vertebrate homolog integrated int-1; ZFP521, zinc-finger protein 521.

blocking activity, but also by decreasing gene expression and protein levels in the posttraumatic joint with OA.

During the past few years, abnormal catabolic activation via some specific receptors has been identified. Transmembrane heparan sulfate proteoglycan syndecan-4 regulates MMP-3 expression by activating ERK1/2 and by controlling the activation of ADAMTS-5 through regulation of mitogen-activated protein kinase.[39] Discoidin domain receptor 2 (DDR2) activation is implicated in the induction and upregulation of MMP-13 in chondrocytes and disruption of the pericellular matrix.[40] Therefore, inhibition of syndecan-4 and/or reduction of DDR2 may also constitute a promising clinical strategy to attenuate the progression of OA.

CHONDROCYTES IN VITRO AND CHONDROGENIC STRATEGY CHOICE

Several strategies are being studied in attempt to prevent loss of the chondrocyte phenotype and subsequent matrix degradation. Emerging data suggest that a combination of different factors may be able to prevent cartilage degeneration. It is well-established that isolated and expanded primary chondrocytes in monolayer culture tend to lose their phenotype with passage of time, because subcultures of differentiated chondrocytes lose their normal rounded, polygonal morphology as they dedifferentiate, assuming an elongated, fibroblast-like morphology with expression of collagen I and III genes instead of collagens II, IX, XI, and aggrecan.[41]

Different factors as well as different culture systems that support chondrocyte phenotype have been widely studied. Various culture systems support the chondrocyte phenotype, including suspension cultures, high cell-seeding density in pellet culture or micromass culture, culture on different types of biomaterials such substrates coated with collagens I and II, agarose, alginate, and hyaluronan hydrogels,[42] and new cell-free scaffold strategies such as biomimetic scaffolds.[43,44] The effects of cell seeding density on slowing the dedifferentiation process has been reported in pig articular chondrocytes.[45] In addition to approaches to delay chondrocyte dedifferentiation, other avenues have been investigated, including culturing under hypoxia,[46] mechanical stimulation, and the effects of growth factor supplementation with TGF-β1 and -3, fibroblast growth factor-2, insulin-like growth factor-1, and bone morphogenic proteins 2 and 7.[47]

Another important consideration is the unique approach of coculturing chondrocytes with mesenchymal stem cells (MSCs). One of the most important challenges in articular cartilage tissue engineering is the choice of the cell types and culture conditions that are most effective for the maintenance or restoration of the differentiated chondrocyte phenotype. MSCs have been a focus of intense in vitro and preclinical (animal) research, and their ability to differentiate into specific lineages, including the chondrogenic lineage, makes them a promising cell source for cartilage repair. Synovium-derived cells are reported to exhibit the greatest chondrogenic potential among the other mesenchymal tissue-derived cells examined.[48,49] However, MSCs chondrogenesis remains challenging, because cells that are differentiated into chondrocytes are typically not able to maintain the chondrocyte phenotype, but rather continue toward chondrocyte hypertrophy, with subsequent matrix mineralization. In an effort to better understand these mechanisms the new approach of coculture of chondrocytes with MSCs has arisen, and it seems that the resultant cell–cell interactions may suppress either MSC hypertrophy or chondrocyte dedifferentiation.[47,50] Nevertheless, the coculturing does not prevent MSC hypertrophy completely or maintain the chondrocyte differentiation status definitively. However, these do seem to be promising strategies and future studies are needed to identify the optimal coculture conditions and to clarify the mechanisms behind these cell–cell interactions and their ECM environments.

RESPONSE TO INJURY: PARTIAL THICKNESS × FULL THICKNESS

Articular cartilage injuries have very limited capacity for self-repair and limited ability of mature chondrocytes to produce a sufficient amount of ECM. Untreated cartilage injuries, therefore, lead to the development of OA. The main reasons for limited capacity to self-repair and regenerate seems to be the avascular nature of cartilage tissue and inability for clot formation, which is the basic step in the healing cascade.[51] That is why progenitor cells in blood and bone marrow and resident chondrocytes are unable to migrate to sites of the articular cartilage lesion. Generally, intrinsic cartilage repair does not follow the main steps that usually occur after an injury in other tissues: necrosis, inflammation, and repair or remodeling. Furthermore, mature chondrocytes have limited proliferative potential and have a limited ability to produce a sufficient amount of ECM to fill a defect. However, several different cell types are mobilized to articular cartilage after an injury and can produce new matrix, although this matrix is morphologically and mechanically inferior to the original native articular cartilage tissue. Articular cartilage injuries can be divided into partial thickness defects, which do not penetrate the subchondral bone and do not repair spontaneously, and full-thickness defects, which penetrate the subchondral bone and have partial repair potential, depending on the size and location of the defect (**Fig. 4**).[52] Partial thickness injuries are commonly encountered in orthopedic surgery. It has been observed that the cells adjacent to the lesion margin undergo cell death. However, there is an increase in cell proliferation, chondrocyte cluster formation, and matrix synthesis, but this process does not repair the defect effectively. It has also been documented that cells from synovium can migrate to the lesion in the presence of growth factors and can fill the defect with regenerative tissue. Yoshioka and colleagues[53] reported that the repair

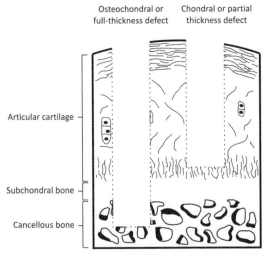

Osteochondral or full-thickness defect   Chondral or partial thickness defect

Articular cartilage

Subchondral bone

Cancellous bone

Fig. 4. Scheme for cartilage injuries. Scheme illustrates a partial thickness focal defect in articular cartilage and a full-thickness defect that penetrates to the subchondral bone. (*Reprinted from* Robi K, Jakob N, Matevz K, et al. Current Issues in Sports and Exercise Medicine. The Physiology of Sports Injuries and Repair Processes Chapter 2. Croatia: InTech; 2013. p. 43–86.)

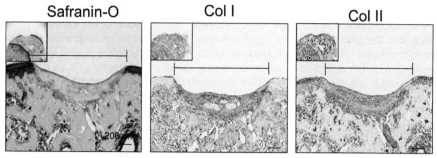

Fig. 5. Cartilage injury in the rat femoral cartilage. Four weeks after full-thickness cartilage injury of 1.5 mm in diameter was created, that defect was filled with fibrous cartilage tissue, negative for safranin-O, positive for type I and type II collagen staining (original magnification, ×100). (*Reprinted from* Nakagawa Y, Muneta T, Otabe K, et al. Cartilage derived from bone marrow mesenchymal stem cells expresses lubricin in vitro and in vivo. PLoS One 2016;11(2):e0148777.)

mechanisms of partial cartilage injury differed according to injury location and orientation in a rabbit model. Better repair was obtained when the injury was parallel to the direction of joint motion rather than perpendicular to joint motion. Recently, analysis of SF after knee injury or in the setting of OA demonstrates a larger number of MSCs compared with normal, healthy knees.[54,55] MSCs from SF might contribute to intrinsic healing of cartilage injuries to some extent. The potential of cartilage repair in full thickness lesions is due to breaching of the subchondral bony plate, which leads to local influx of blood and MSCs and hematoma formation containing fibrin clot, with accumulation of platelets, red cells, and white blood cells. Full-thickness cartilage defects smaller than 3 mm in diameter in a rabbit model reportedly regenerates spontaneously. However, mobilized cells in the newly formatted blood clot are not capable to regenerate native hyaline cartilage, but produce fibrocartilage tissue, composed of a higher collagen type I to collagen type II ratio and less proteoglycan, which has inferior material properties compared with native hyaline cartilage (**Fig. 5**). Several surgical techniques use the same attempt to treat full-thickness defects, including microfracture that penetrates the subchondral bone to stimulate clot formation and to mobilize cells to the site of the cartilage lesion.

Although promising new therapeutic strategies have been developed and tested in preclinical models, autologous chondrocyte implantation is still the only cell-based treatment with approval from the US Food and Drug Administration.[56] These techniques are still not able to fully restore the tissue, producing fibrocartilage repair tissue, which is inferior to hyaline cartilage for the intended purposes of load bearing and joint movement. Thus, new cell-based and tissue engineering approaches are necessary and continue to be evaluated and optimized with the aim of promoting and inducing cartilage regeneration.

SUMMARY

The most challenging aspects in the treatment of articular cartilage injury include identifying the cellular and molecular mechanism(s) that lead to matrix changes and the differentiation and dedifferentiation behavior of chondrocytes, and understanding how they affect the structural integrity of the articular cartilage and eventual tissue remodeling. In recent years, several biological treatment strategies including stem cell approaches and scaffold technologies have been proposed to provide less invasive and more effective cartilage repair. A better understanding of the signaling pathways, and the growth and transcription factors for specific genes responsible for the chondrogenesis process, which involves chondrocyte differentiation and maturation resulting in cartilage and bone formation during skeletal development, is an important component in the development of new therapies that either prevent cartilage degeneration or promote repair to replicate the physiologic and functional properties of the original cartilage.

REFERENCES

1. Johnstone B, Alini M, Cucchiarini M, et al. Tissue engineering for articular cartilage repair—the state of the art. Eur Cell Mater 2013;25:248–67.
2. Musumeci G, Loreto C, Imbesi R, et al. Advantages of exercise in rehabilitation, treatment and prevention of altered morphological features in knee osteoarthritis. A narrative review. Histol Histopathol 2014;29(6):707–19.
3. Mow VC, Guo XE. Mechano-electrochemical properties of articular cartilage: their inhomogeneities and anisotropies. Annu Rev Biomed Eng 2002;4:175–209.
4. Brocklehurst R, Bayliss MT, Maroudas A, et al. The composition of normal and osteoarthritic articular cartilage from Tissue Engineering Zonal Cartilage human knee joints. With special reference to unicompartmental replacement and osteotomy of the knee. J Bone Joint Surg Am 1984;66:95–106.
5. Nakagawa Y, Muneta T, Otabe K, et al. Cartilage derived from bone marrow mesenchymal stem cells expresses lubricin in vitro and in vivo. PLoS One 2016;11(2):e0148777.
6. Ateshian GA, Warden WH, Kim JJ, et al. Finite deformation biphasic material properties of bovine articular cartilage from confined compression experiments. J Biomech 1997;30:1157–64.
7. Mow VC, Ateshian GA, Ratcliffe A. Anatomic form and biomechanical properties of articular cartilage of the knee joint. In: Finerman GAM, Noyes FR, editors. Biology and biomechanics of the traumatized synovial joint: the knee as a model. 2nd edition. Washington, DC: American Academy of Orthopaedic Surgeons; 1993.
8. Mankin HJ, Mow VC, Buckwalter JA, et al. Form and function of articular cartilage. Rosemont (IL): American Academy of Orthopaedic Surgeons; 1992. p. 55–81.
9. Simon SR, editor. Orthopaedic basic science. Rosemont (IL): American Academy of Orthopaedic Surgeons; 1994. p. 1–44.
10. Maroudas A. Physiochemical properties of articular cartilage. In: Freeman MAR, editor. Adult articular cartilage. Kent (United Kingdom): Cambridge University Press; 1979. p. 215–90.
11. Frank EH, Grodzinsky AJ. Cartilage electromechanics: I. Electrokinetic transduction and the effects of electrolyte pH and ionic strength. J Biomech 1987;20: 615–27.
12. Schmidt TA, Gastelum NS, Nguyen QT, et al. Boundary lubrication of articular cartilage: role of synovial fluid constituents. Arthritis Rheum 2007;56(3):882–91.
13. Daniel M. Boundary cartilage lubrication: review of current concepts [review]. Wien Med Wochenschr 2014;164(5–6):88–94.
14. Zelenski NA, Leddy HA, Sanchez-Adams J, et al. Type VI collagen regulates pericellular matrix properties, chondrocyte swelling, and mechanotransduction in mouse articular cartilage. Arthritis Rheumatol 2015;67(5):1286–94.

15. Eyre DR, Weis MA, Wu JJ. Articular cartilage collagen: an irreplaceable framework? Eur Cell Mater 2006;12:57–63.
16. Culav EM, Clark CH, Merrilees MJ. Connective tissues: matrix composition and its relevance to physical therapy. Phys Ther 1999;79(3):308–19.
17. Brody LT. Knee osteoarthritis: clinical connections to articular cartilage structure and function. Phys Ther Sport 2015;16(4):301–16.
18. Roughley PJ. Articular cartilage and changes in arthritis: noncollagenous proteins and proteoglycans in the extracellular matrix of cartilage. Arthritis Res 2001;3(6): 342–7.
19. Melrose J, Fuller ES, Roughley PJ, et al. Fragmentation of decorin, biglycan, lumican and keratocan is elevated in degenerate human meniscus, knee and hip articular cartilages compared with age-matched macroscopically normal and control tissues. Arthritis Res Ther 2008;10(4):R79.
20. Costell M, Gustafsson E, Aszódi A, et al. Perlecan maintains the integrity of cartilage and some basement membranes. J Cell Biol 1999;147(5):1109–22.
21. Sadatsuki R, Kaneko H, Kinoshita M, et al. Perlecan is required for the chondrogenic differentiation of synovial mesenchymal cells through regulation of Sox9 gene expression. J Orthop Res 2016. http://dx.doi.org/10.1002/jor.23318.
22. Flannery CR, Hughes CE, Schumacher BL, et al. Articular cartilage superficial zone protein (SZP) is homologous to megakaryocyte stimulating factor precursor and Is a multifunctional proteoglycan with potential growth-promoting, cytoprotective, and lubricating properties in cartilage metabolism. Biochem Biophys Res Commun 1999;254(3):535–41.
23. Ulrich-Vinther M, Maloney MD, Schwarz EM, et al. Articular cartilage biology. J Am Acad Orthop Surg 2003;11(6):421–30.
24. Kozhemyakina E, Lassar AB, Zelzer E. A pathway to bone: signaling molecules and transcription factors involved in chondrocyte development and maturation. Development 2015;142(5):817–31.
25. Goldring MB, Tsuchimochi K, Ijiri K. The control of chondrogenesis. J Cell Biochem 2006;97(1):33–44.
26. Goldring MB, Otero M. Inflammation in osteoarthritis. Curr Opin Rheumatol 2011; 23(5):471–8.
27. Loeser RF. Molecular mechanisms of cartilage destruction: mechanics, inflammatory mediators, and aging collide. Arthritis Rheum 2006;54(5):1357–60.
28. Tsuchida AI, Beekhuizen M, 't Hart MC, et al. Cytokine profiles in the joint depend on pathology, but are different between synovial fluid, cartilage tissue and cultured chondrocytes. Arthritis Res Ther 2014;16(5):441.
29. Klatt AR, Paul-Klausch B, Klinger G, et al. A critical role for collagen II in cartilage matrix degradation: collagen II induces pro-inflammatory cytokines and MMPs in primary human chondrocytes. J Orthop Res 2009;27(1):65–70.
30. Joosten LA, Smeets RL, Koenders MI, et al. Interleukin-18 promotes joint inflammation and induces interleukin-1-driven cartilage destruction. Am J Pathol 2004; 165(3):959–67.
31. Zhen G, Wen C, Jia X, et al. Inhibition of TGF-β signaling in mesenchymal stem cells of subchondral bone attenuates osteoarthritis. Nat Med 2013;19(6):704–12.
32. Handorf AM, Chamberlain CS, Li WJ. Endogenously produced Indian hedgehog regulates TGFβ-driven chondrogenesis of human bone marrow stromal/stem cells. Stem Cells Dev 2014;24:995–1007.
33. Rengel Y, Ospelt C, Gay S. Proteinases in the joint: clinical relevance of proteinases in joint destruction. Arthritis Res Ther 2007;9(5):221.

34. Little CB, Barai A, Burkhardt D, et al. Matrix metalloproteinase 13-deficient mice are resistant to osteoarthritic cartilage erosion but not chondrocyte hypertrophy or osteophyte development. Arthritis Rheum 2009;60(12):3723–33.

35. Leong DJ, Li YH, Gu XI, et al. Physiological loading of joints prevents cartilage degradation through CITED2. FASEB J 2011;25(1):182–91.

36. Otero M, Plumb DA, Tsuchimochi K, et al. E74-like factor 3 (ELF3) impacts on matrix metalloproteinase 13 (MMP13) transcriptional control in articular chondrocytes under proinflammatory stress. J Biol Chem 2012;287(5):3559–72.

37. Olivotto E, Otero M, Astolfi A, et al. IKKα/CHUK regulates extracellular matrix remodeling independent of its kinase activity to facilitate articular chondrocyte differentiation. PLoS One 2013;8(9):e73024.

38. Wang S, Wei X, Zhou J, et al. Identification of α2-macroglobulin as a master inhibitor of cartilage-degrading factors that attenuates the progression of posttraumatic osteoarthritis. Arthritis Rheumatol 2014;66(7):1843–53.

39. Echtermeyer F, Bertrand J, Dreier R, et al. Syndecan-4 regulates ADAMTS-5 activation and cartilage breakdown in osteoarthritis. Nat Med 2009;15(9):1072–6.

40. Xu L, Servais J, Polur I, et al. Attenuation of osteoarthritis progression by reduction of discoidin domain receptor 2 in mice. Arthritis Rheum 2010;62(9):2736–44.

41. Gosset M, Berenbaum F, Thirion S, et al. Primary culture and phenotyping of murine chondrocytes. Nat Protoc 2008;3(8):1253–60.

42. Otero M, Favero M, Dragomir C, et al. Human chondrocyte cultures as models of cartilage-specific gene regulation. Methods Mol Biol 2012;806:301–36.

43. Berruto M, Delcogliano M, de Caro F, et al. Treatment of large knee osteochondral lesions with a biomimetic scaffold: results of a multicenter study of 49 patients at 2-year follow-up. Am J Sports Med 2014;42(7):1607–17.

44. Samaroo KJ, Tan M, Putnam D, et al. Binding and lubrication of biomimetic boundary lubricants on articular cartilage. J Orthop Res 2016. http://dx.doi.org/10.1002/jor.23370.

45. Watt FM. Effect of seeding density on stability of the differentiated phenotype of pig articular chondrocytes in culture. J Cell Sci 1988;89(Pt3):373–8.

46. Foldager CB, Nielsen AB, Munir S, et al. Combined 3D and hypoxic culture improves cartilage-specific gene expression in human chondrocytes. Acta Orthop 2011;82(2):234–40.

47. Nazempour A, Van Wie BJ. Chondrocytes, mesenchymal stem cells, and their combination in articular cartilage regenerative medicine. Ann Biomed Eng 2016;44(5):1325–54.

48. Sakaguchi Y, Sekiya I, Yagishita K, et al. Comparison of human stem cells derived from various mesenchymal tissues: superiority of synovium as a cell source. Arthritis Rheum 2005;52(8):2521–9.

49. Shirasawa S, Sekiya I, Sakaguchi Y, et al. In vitro chondrogenesis of human synovium-derived mesenchymal stem cells: optimal condition and comparison with bone marrow-derived cells. J Cell Biochem 2006;97(1):84–97.

50. Hubka KM, Dahlin RL, Meretoja VV, et al. Enhancing chondrogenic phenotype for cartilage tissue engineering: monoculture and coculture of articular chondrocytes and mesenchymal stem cells. Tissue Eng Part B Rev 2014;20(6):641–54.

51. Mow VC, Rosenwasser M. Articular cartilage: biomechanics. In: Woo SL-Y, Buckwalter JA, editors. Injury and repair to the musculoskeletal soft tissues. Park Ridge (IL): American Academy of Orthopaedic Surgeons; 1988. p. 427–46.

52. Redman SN, Oldfield SF, Archer CW. Current strategies for articular cartilage repair. Eur Cell Mater 2005;9:23–32.

53. Yoshioka M, Kubo T, Coutts RD, et al. Differences in the repair process of longitudinal and transverse injuries of cartilage in the rat knee. Osteoarthritis Cartilage 1998;6:66–75.
54. Morito T, Muneta T, Hara K, et al. Synovial fluid-derived mesenchymal stem cells increase after intra-articular ligament injury in humans. Rheumatology (Oxford) 2008;47:1137–43.
55. Sekiya I, Ojima M, Suzuki S, et al. Human mesenchymal stem cells in synovial fluid increase in the knee with degenerated cartilage and osteoarthritis. J Orthop Res 2012;30:943–9.
56. Hwang NS, Elisseeff J. Application of stem cells for articular cartilage regeneration. J Knee Surg 2009;22(1):60–71.

Imaging of Cartilage in the Athlete

Christopher M. Coleman, MD*, Jonathan A. Flug, MD, MBA, Nancy Major, MD

KEYWORDS

- MRI • Cartilage injury • Cartilage repair

KEY POINTS

- MRI is the optimal test for identification of cartilage injuries and for evaluating these patients after cartilage repair surgery.
- Standard MRI evaluation allows for a morphologic cartilage evaluation addressing the cartilage thickness, intrinsic cartilage signal, and subchondral bone.
- Compositional MRI techniques specifically quantify the quantity of particular molecules within the extracellular cartilage matrix and may allow for an earlier diagnosis of cartilage injury before morphologic changes manifest.

INTRODUCTION

Articular cartilage lesions represent a growing class of injuries in collegiate, professional, and recreational athletes with limited intrinsic healing capacity.[1] Due to the prevalence of these injuries and their associated sequela, diagnosis with noninvasive imaging modalities is extremely helpful to be able to appropriately treat these patients and determine their long-term prognosis. This article discusses imaging of cartilage injuries in athletes and the imaging of surgical cartilage repair techniques, with an emphasis on MRI.

MRI remains the ideal imaging technique for evaluation of articular cartilage, as it allows for direct visualization of the cartilage and the subchondral bone. MRI uses nonionizing radiation and therefore avoids the associated health risks caused by ionizing radiation, which is particularly relevant for this class of injuries that may involve younger patients with multiple imaging studies. MRI is also ideal because it can be obtained in multiple planes and provides exquisite soft tissue contrast. Additionally, MRI provides an ideal evaluation of the other soft tissue structures around the joint that may be injured. Radiographs and computed tomography (CT) provide an evaluation of the cartilage indirectly by evaluating the joint space thickness and associated

Disclosure Statement: The authors have no relevant disclosures related to the work.
Department of Radiology, University of Colorado Hospital, 12605 East 16th Avenue, Aurora, CO 80045, USA
* Corresponding author.
E-mail address: Christopher.m.coleman@ucdenver.edu

Clin Sports Med 36 (2017) 427–445
http://dx.doi.org/10.1016/j.csm.2017.02.002
0278-5919/17/© 2017 Elsevier Inc. All rights reserved.

sportsmed.theclinics.com

bone changes, but have limited ability to directly visualize the cartilage tissue. Contrast arthrography using radiographs and CT allow for a more detailed evaluation of the cartilage surface, but still do not provide the same level of detail that MRI provides when evaluating the cartilage tissue and include the risks associated with ionizing radiation.

Although MRI is the ideal imaging examination in patients suspected of having an articular cartilage injury, this modality can be contraindicated, particularly when the patient has a pacemaker or other implanted medical device that is not safe for MRI. In these cases, alternative examinations, such as CT arthrography, may be able to provide adequate evaluation of the cartilage. Direct consultation with a radiologist is helpful in these situations to determine the most appropriate alternative imaging modality.

MRI evaluation using standard sequences provides high-resolution, high-contrast techniques that will allow for imaging in multiple planes, yet also be completed in a timely fashion. Technological advances in MRI have led to the development of a variety of imaging techniques that allow for a compositional evaluation of the articular cartilage, which can potentially evaluate molecular changes to the cartilage before morphologic changes, including techniques such as delayed gadolinium-enhanced MRI of cartilage (dGEMRIC), T2 mapping, and T1 rho. Adequate evaluation of the articular cartilage requires high–spatial resolution imaging because of the small thickness of articular cartilage, with imaging performed in 3 orthogonal planes. High resolution is accomplished by the use of a surface coil over the joint of interest. Field strengths of 1.5 T can generally provide adequate signal for morphologic evaluation of the articular cartilage. MRI units with 3.0-T field strengths allow for improved signal to noise ratio (SNR), thereby allowing for higher spatial resolution and shorter imaging times. Use of 3.0-T MRI has shown higher diagnostic accuracy compared with 1.5 T for the evaluation of cartilage in the knee.[2] A field strength of at least 1.0 T is recommended for cartilage evaluation and field strengths of 0.20 T have been shown to be inadequate to reliably evaluate cartilage.[3,4] Limitations of 3.0-T units include increased metallic susceptibility artifact compared with 1.5 T, particularly in the postoperative patient or patient with implanted hardware.

When evaluating articular cartilage, the normal hyaline cartilage will demonstrate an intermediate signal with a trilaminar pattern of stratification on T2-weighted or proton density (PD)-weighted sequences (**Fig. 1**). The surface layer of cartilage should have low signal intensity, the intermediate layer should have high signal intensity, and the deep layer should have low signal intensity. This is often most evident in thicker cartilage, such as the patellar cartilage.[5] The signal pattern in each layer of cartilage remains related to the orientation of collagen fibrils in that layer and the distribution of chondrocytes.

MORPHOLOGIC CARTILAGE EVALUATION

The sequence selection needs to provide adequate soft tissue contrast to differentiate between the joint fluid and cartilage along with differentiation between the cartilage and the subchondral bone. Attention should be paid to the intrinsic signal within the cartilage, the presence of fissuring, and the presence of partial-thickness or full-thickness cartilage loss. The presence of fibrillation or irregularity of cartilage surface should be addressed. Focal fissuring is identified, as focal linear or wedge-shaped regions of increased signal extending to the lamina splendens. Focal cartilage damage should be described as either partial thickness or full thickness extending to the

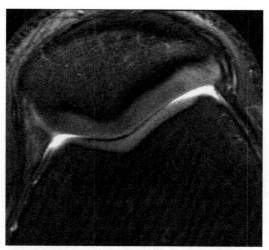

Fig. 1. Axial PD fat suppressed (FS)-weighted image demonstrating normal patellar and trochlear cartilage with intermediate signal.

subchondral bone. Any associated subchondral marrow edema, cystic change, or sclerosis can provide information about chronicity of injury and quality of the remaining cartilage. If linear high signal extends into the underlying marrow, an osteochondral lesion (OCL) should be suspected. If this signal extends in an arc and violates the articular surface in 2 places, or if intra-articular gadolinium completely undercuts the lesion, it should be considered likely unstable (**Fig. 2**).

Grading of cartilage lesions is often performed using a modified Noyes or Outerbridge Scale, corresponding to the arthroscopic grading of these lesions, although arthroscopy remains the gold standard for diagnosis of cartilage lesions[6] (**Fig. 3**, **Table 1**). The International Cartilage Repair Society Classification is another commonly used grading system. Grading is controversial, as correlation is poor between magnetic resonance (MR) grading and arthroscopic grading.[7]

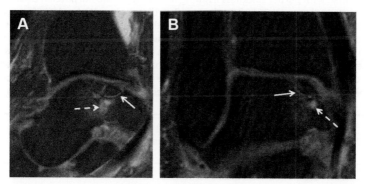

Fig. 2. Sagittal (*A*) and coronal (*B*) PD FS-weighted images of the ankle in a 56-year-old woman with ankle pain. There is an osteochondral lesion involving the superomedial talar dome. Fluid signal completely undercuts the lesion with adjacent sclerosis (*solid arrow*) along with cystic change along the margins of the lesions (*dashed arrow*) consistent with an unstable osteochondral lesion.

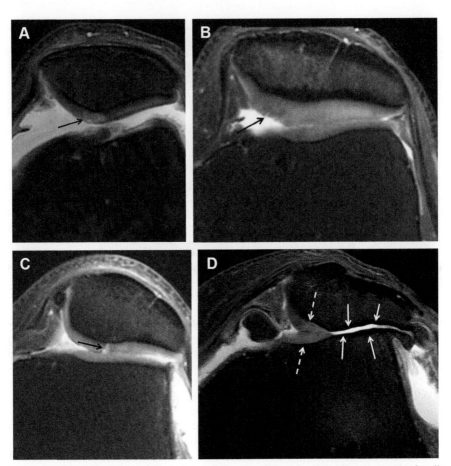

Fig. 3. (*A*) Axial PD FS image in a 47-year-old man with knee pain demonstrating focally increased signal within the patellar cartilage at the apex (*black arrow*) consistent with softening, corresponding to an Outerbridge grade 1 cartilage injury. (*B*) Axial PD FS image in a 33-year-old man with partial-thickness fissuring involving the medial patellar cartilage (*black arrow*), corresponding to an Outerbridge grade 2 cartilage injury. (*C*) Axial PD FS image in a 28-year-old man with a full-thickness fissure involving the lateral patellar cartilage that extends to the subchondral bone (*black arrow*), corresponding to an Outerbridge grade 3 cartilage injury. (*D*) Axial PD FS image in a 40-year-old woman with full-thickness cartilage loss extending to the subchondral bone involving the lateral patellar facet and lateral trochlea (*white arrows*), corresponding to an Outerbridge grade 4 cartilage injury. There is persistent partial-thickness cartilage involving the medial patella and trochlea (*dashed arrows*).

Table 1
Outerbridge grading scale

Grade	Features
0	Normal-appearing cartilage
1	Soft, swollen cartilage
2	Partial-thickness defect, or diameter <1.5 cm
3	Fissures that extend to the subchondral surface with diameter >1.5 cm
4	Exposed subchondral bone

A technique that is largely used for cartilage evaluation is fast spin echo (FSE) imaging, particularly intermediate or PD-weighted sequences. Traditional T1-weighted images do not adequately differentiate cartilage from the adjacent synovial fluid (**Fig. 4**) and T2-weighted sequences do not adequately differentiate cartilage from subchondral bone, making it difficult to accurately identify cartilage defects, including thin fissures and delamination. PD-weighted sequences provide optimal differentiation between cartilage and subchondral bone. Chemical fat-suppression techniques can be used to increase the conspicuity of marrow abnormalities that can help identify associated cartilage injuries, as well as provide a fluid-sensitive sequence that can help identify the different appearance of cartilage abnormalities. Because hyaline cartilage abnormalities commonly occur in conjunction with fibrocartilaginous (ie, meniscal) and ligamentous pathology, PD-weighted FSE sequences should be part of every joint imaging protocol.

Dual-echo steady-state (DESS), a type of gradient imaging, can be performed in either 2-dimensional (2D) or 3D acquisition. The latter results in high SNR, decreased imaging time, and improved contrast between cartilage and fluid compared with the former.[8] Cartilage remains intermediate in signal, as in FSE T2, while fluid is hyperintense, but with shorter imaging times compared with FSE T2.[9] Gradient-echo imaging is limited in postoperative cases, as accentuated susceptibility artifact can preclude evaluation of cartilage.

MR arthrography can assist in the evaluation of cartilage injuries in select scenarios. Direct MR arthrography is performed by injecting dilute gadolinium contrast into the joint, followed by the MR examination. Generally, multiplanar T1-weighted images with fat saturation and PD-weighted images are subsequently performed. The hyperintense joint fluid caused by the gadolinium will provide excellent contrast to the intermediate-signal cartilage and the hypointense subchondral bone (**Fig. 5**). The intra-articular injection of anesthetics with the contrast can also provide additional diagnostic information, as pain relief with injection confirms an intra-articular pain generator. As the spatial resolution of MRI continues to improve, the need for MR arthrography for cartilage evaluation continues to diminish, particularly in the larger joints.[10]

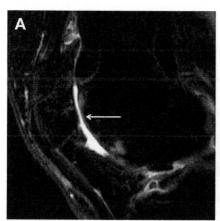 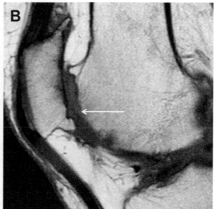

Fig. 4. Sagittal T2 FS (*A*) and sagittal T1-weighted image (*B*) in the same patient demonstrate full-thickness cartilage loss along the patella with partial-thickness cartilage loss in the trochlea (*white arrow*). The degree of cartilage loss is difficult to assess in the T1-weighted image due to the similar signal intensity between cartilage and the surrounding fluid.

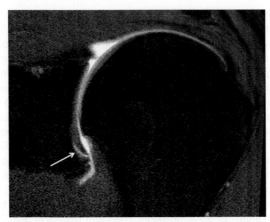

Fig. 5. A coronal T1 FS-weighted image of the shoulder obtained after the intra-articular administration of gadolinium contrast demonstrates a delaminating cartilage flap in the inferior glenoid cartilage (*arrow*).

JOINT-SPECIFIC EVALUATION

Although there are a variety of different mechanisms and patterns of cartilage injury in the knee, one of particular import is the transient patellar dislocation. Retinacular and medial patellofemoral ligament injury are usually readily apparent on MRI. However, impaction injury to either the medial patellar or lateral femoral trochlea cartilage/underlying subchondral bone can be subtle. Identifying the lesions is crucial, as displaced chondral or osteochondral fragments can cause continued pain and lead to early-onset osteoarthritis. Cartilage-sensitive sequences can identify the cartilage defect and often the displaced intra-articular fragment. Recognizing a chondral abnormality will often result in surgical evaluation. Fat-suppressed, fluid-sensitive sequences can identify the underlying marrow edema typically found at the lateral femoral condyle and/or the medial margin of the patella.

OCL (also known as osteochondritis dissecans), is an acquired lesion of subchondral bone involving resorption, sclerosis, fragmentation, or a combination thereof, that can become unstable and ultimately break off, becoming an intra-articular loose body. It should be differentiated from an osteochondral fracture.

In situ fixation with Herbert screws, Kirschner wires, and other devices also can be used to stabilize these lesions. The general consensus is to use in situ fixation for lesions occupying less than 50% of the articular surface.

The capitellum is a common location for OCL in young athletic adults, particularly those with repetitive overhead motion. A variety of treatment strategies have been proposed, ranging from rest to chondroplasty, microfracture, fragment fixation, osteochondral autograft transfer (OAT), and allograft procedures, as well as arthroscopic removal of loose bodies.[11]

MRI of early capitellar OCL demonstrates subarticular low T1 signal, followed by increased T2. A thin rim of high T2 signal around the lesion or immediately subjacent cystic changes are associated with instability at arthroscopy.[12]

Conservative management is appropriate for stable lesions in most cases. Surgical intervention is indicated for those with MRI and clinical evidence of lesion instability, including fluid signal encircling the fragment, or in those who have failed conservative management.[13]

Abrasion chondroplasty and loose body removal without reconstruction is useful in select cases, especially when less than 50% of capitellum articular surface is involved, and the lesion does not extend into the lateral capitellum.[11,14]

The incidence of Outerbridge grade II-IV lesions in the glenohumeral joint is estimated at 5% during arthroscopic evaluation.[15] These may be related to a wide spectrum of pathology, including idiopathic focal defects, chondrolysis, posttraumatic defects, OCL, avascular necrosis, postsurgical cartilage abnormalities, and osteoarthritis. Cartilage injuries in particular are seen in acute and recurrent cases of shoulder instability. Although shoulder arthroplasty represents a successful surgical technique for many of these patients, it poses a challenge providing optimal long-term outcomes in the young, active patient with symptomatic cartilage loss.[16] One common mechanism is a shearing injury as can be seen with overhead motion. The articular cartilage can be sheared at the level of the tidemark from the underlying bone. This can lead to delamination.

Cartilage injuries in the hip joint may arise from a variety of pathologic processes, including femoroacetabular impingement, acetabular dysplasia, trauma, and avascular necrosis. Again, the mechanism is often a shear-type injury. Articular cartilage injuries can be graded using the Outerbridge classification, as well as the Beck classification and the Acetabular Labrum Articular Disruption classification.[17,18] Open surgical hip dislocation and hip arthroscopy allow for implementation of many of the cartilage surgical repair techniques described previously.

BIOLOGICAL OPTIONS FOR CARTILAGE REPAIR

MRI can provide an evaluation of the morphologic and compositional quality of the repaired cartilage and associated bone using the techniques described previously, which may provide important information about the status of the repair and the possibility of further cartilage injury. Understanding the physiology of the repair technique and the stage of healing are critical to be able to appropriately evaluate the postprocedural imaging. The MR Observations of Cartilage Repair Tissue (MOCART) scoring system has excellent interobserver reproducibility for scoring of the defined variables, and it is an effective method for standardized reporting of the imaging features of autologous chondrocyte implants (ACIs). The parameters that can be evaluated with MR imaging at *microfracture sites* and *osteochondral autograft transplant* sites include the degree of defect filling, the extent of integration of repair tissue with adjacent tissues, the presence or absence of proud subchondral bone formation (extension of repair tissue beyond the adjacent subchondral plate to include new bone formation), the characteristics of the graft substance and surface, the appearance of the underlying bone, and the cartilage adjacent to the repair.[19,20]

Standard morphologic MR evaluation of cartilage repair should be performed on a 1.5-T or 3.0-T scanner to achieve the necessary spatial resolution in reasonable scan times. Morphologic MR evaluation can be performed using the standard cartilage imaging techniques, including intermediate-weighted FSE sequences and 3D fat-suppressed T1-weighted gradient-echo (GRE) acquisition. The FSE sequence is more sensitive for assessment of the intrinsic cartilage signal, whereas the GRE sequence is suitable for cartilage thickness and surface contour evaluation.[20]

Microfracture and Enhanced Microfracture

Microfracture, along with abrasion arthroplasty and subchondral drilling, are mechanical techniques used to perforate the subchondral plate of bone. The resultant hematoma extends into the damaged cartilage bringing growth factors and cytokines to the cartilage defect and inciting a healing cascade. It is currently regarded by many as the gold standard for cartilage repair.[21] One limitation of microfracture, however, is that the fibrocartilage that is ultimately generated is suboptimal compared with the native hyaline cartilage in its ability to absorb and distribute force. Many think that this contributes to later deterioration following initial improvement of symptomatology.[22,23]

The postoperative appearance of lesions treated with microfracture evolve over time. Initially, the repair tissue may appear thin and indistinct, but within 1 to 2 years the reparative tissue should fill the defect, and should appear smooth and well defined (**Fig. 6**). The signal intensity of the reparative tissue will initially be relatively hyperintense to the adjacent cartilage related to the less organized matrix and increased mobility of water within the tissue. As the tissue matures, the intrinsic cartilage signal and subchondral bone marrow edema should decrease. Persistent bone marrow edema and incomplete filling of the defect with thin and irregular repair tissue are indicative of treatment failure (**Figs. 7** and **8**).[19,20]

An additional proposed contributor to eventual failure after microfracture is osseous overgrowth of the subchondral bone. This overgrowth, also known as intralesional osteophytosis, can thin the overlying reparative cartilage and possibly alter biomechanics, leading to eventual treatment failure. On MRI, subchondral bony overgrowth is best identified on intermediate-weighted FSE sequences, and appears as tissue isointense to cancellous bone in the region of the microfracture, extending into the cartilage defect (**Fig. 9**).[24] Osseous overgrowth has been seen in most cases, and significantly increased risk of failure (25% vs 3%) compared with those without overgrowth.[25]

Radiologists and orthopedic surgeons alike who interpret MRI after cartilage treatment need to evaluate for these potential findings. The appearance is the same in all joints, as microfracture has been used in locations beyond the knee joint (**Fig. 10**).

Osteochondral Autograft

OAT is one of the original surgical techniques for treating cartilage lesions. It involves taking mature hyaline cartilage and underlying subchondral bone from a remote site, often a non–weight-bearing surface, and using it to fill in the void created by the chondral lesion. Complications include donor site morbidity, lack of incorporation along the articular surface, and accelerated perilesional chondromalacia.

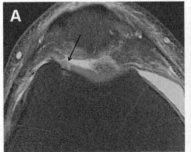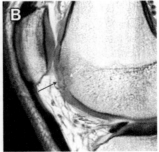

Fig. 6. Axial PD FS (*A*) and sagittal PD-weighted (*B*) images of a 29-year-old man 7 years postoperative from a lateral patellar dislocation and microfracture of the lateral trochlea. There is very minimal persistent subchondral edema and evidence of prior drilling (*black* and *white arrows*). There is mildly heterogeneous signal within the tissue filling the lateral trochlea gap that closely approximates that of the native cartilage.

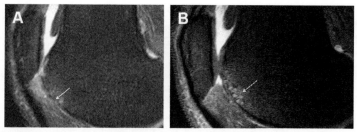

Fig. 7. Sagittal PD FS before (*A*) and 5 years after (*B*) lateral femoral condyle microfracture shows cartilage loss in the lateral trochlea (*white arrow*). The patient had persistent pain and was imaged demonstrating minimal fibrocartilage fill with significant progression of the bone marrow edema and development of subchondral cystic change indicative of treatment failure (*broken arrow*).

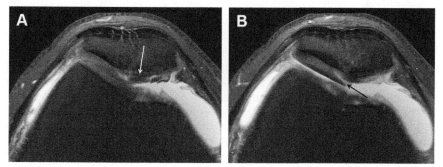

Fig. 8. Axial PD FS images in a 23-year-old man with prior microfracture repair at the patellar apex. There is partial fibrocartilage fill involving the cartilage defect (*A*) (*white arrow*). Despite the repair, there is a delaminating cartilage flap involving the lateral patellar cartilage (*B*) (*black arrow*) that has progressed since the pre-procedural images.

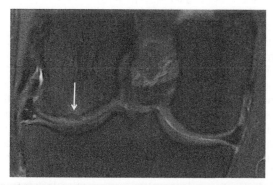

Fig. 9. Coronal PD FS image in a patient post microfracture in the lateral femoral condyle shows osseous overgrowth involving the subchondral bone (*white arrow*). The repair tissue remains congruent with the adjacent cartilage.

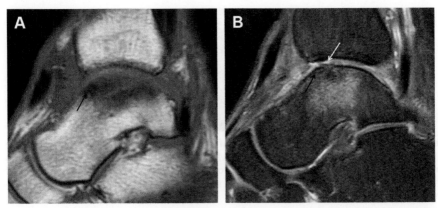

Fig. 10. Sagittal T1-weighted (*A*) and PD FS (*B*) images of the left ankle after having undergone multiple prior surgeries including talar dome microfracture and prior cartilage grafting. There is subchondral sclerosis (*black arrow*) and subjacent edema. The talar dome articular surface is flattened with full-thickness cartilage loss (*white arrow*) consistent with procedure failure.

Imaging in the postoperative state should focus on the degree of defect filling by the plug, the marginal integration of the cartilage and bone, the cartilage surface contour, and the intrinsic signal within the bone plug. Expected findings include associated marrow edema in the native bone and increased T2 signal in the donor bone and cartilage layer. This should improve over the course of a year on follow-up imaging studies. The cleft between the donor and recipient cartilage implant should obscure over time as well. Any new edemalike signal in the donor cartilage, increased cortical bone signal in the graft, or new protrusion of the graft beyond the margins of the recipient site should prompt concern for failure.[26] Link and colleagues[27] reported no significant correlation between clinical and MRI findings in patients undergoing osteochondral autografts, and in particular, no consistent findings in the cases of autograft necrosis.

The OAT procedure has been used in joints in addition to the knee with similar MRI appearances of incorporation or failure.

Osteochondral Allograft

Osteochondral allografts have gained popularity in recent years, due in part to improved standards for storage and regulation. Although generally indicated for lesions larger than 2 cm^2, they demonstrate great versatility of utility, as they can be configured to a wide variety of lesions, including those with irregular margins and those in peripheral locations. The procedure is single stage, and can be used for osteochondral or simply chondral lesions.

Non–fat-suppressed T1-weighted or PD-weighted MRI and plain radiographs can be useful to demonstrate osseous incorporation of the graft, as the fatty marrow can readily be assessed extending into the graft. Fat-suppressed images can make evaluation of incorporation more difficult. Expected postoperative imaging findings include early bone marrow edema within the graft, which decreases within 3 to 6 months (**Fig. 11**). Persistent bone marrow edema beyond 12 months, fluid signal intensity at the graft-host interface, eburnation, osteophytosis, or surface collapse may be indicative of graft rejection or incomplete incorporation.[19,20,28] Subchondral cystic change is also associated with graft failure (**Figs. 12–14**). CT arthrogram can be performed for graft evaluation if MRI is contraindicated (**Fig. 15**). Failed incorporation is

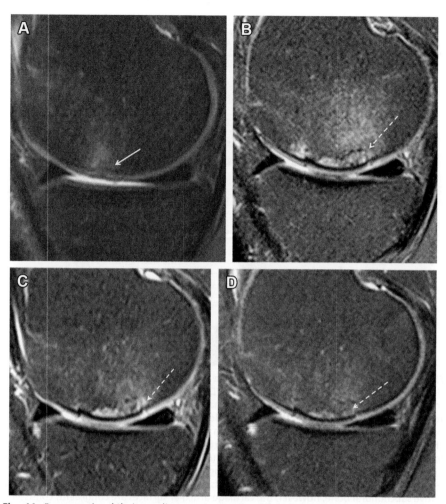

Fig. 11. Preoperative (*A*), immediate postoperative (*B*), 10-month postoperative (*C*), and 13-month postoperative (*D*) sagittal PD FS images in a 43-year-old man shows an osteochondral lesion in the medial femoral condyle (*white arrow*) with subsequent osteochondral allograft placement. The sequential images demonstrate edema in the graft and subchondral bone that decreases over time with progressive osseous incorporation of the graft (*dashed arrows* in *B–D*). Arthroscopy was performed confirming the stability of the graft.

thought to be biomechanical, rather than immunogenic, as evidenced by histochemical analysis.[29]

Autologous Chondrocytes and Next-Generation Matrix-Based Autologous Chondrocyte Implantation

Cell therapy, an important part of cartilage lesion treatment, includes using chondrocytes to stimulate a person's body to generate its own reparative tissue. The original procedure involved direct chondrocyte implantation. The current iteration of this technology involves matrix-applied characterized autologous cultured chondrocytes (MACI; Genzyme Biosurgery, Cambridge, MA) implantation. The current generation produces less osseous hypertrophy than previous techniques.[30]

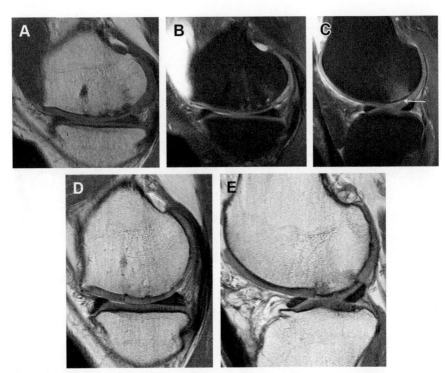

Fig. 12. A 37-year-old man 1 year postoperative from a medial femoral condyle osteochondral allograft. Sagittal T1-weighted (*A*) and PD FS-weighted images (*B*) demonstrate an incorporating graft with minimal marrow edema. Sagittal PD FS images through the lateral femoral condyle (*C*) demonstrate cartilage delamination with underlying subchondral edema (*white arrow*). The patient underwent a subsequent lateral femoral condyle osteochondral allograft. Follow-up imaging was performed 5 years later. Sagittal PD-weighted image through the medial femoral condyle (*D*) demonstrates a continued satisfactory appearance of the medial femoral condyle allograft. Sagittal PD-weighted image through the lateral femoral condyle (*E*) shows slight offset of the osseous portion of the graft and native subchondral bone; however, the cartilage articular surfaces are congruent, consistent with a satisfactory appearance.

MRI can be used to assess the fill of the cartilage defect by reparative tissue using the Whole Organ MRI score (WORMS), which uses a quartile-based grading scale,[31] or the MOCART system.[32] Ideal integration leads to a continuous margin between the native cartilage and the repair without discernable interface. Initially, the repair tissue will demonstrate hyperintense signal that should decrease over time and ultimately approach similar signal intensity to the native adjacent cartilage. Persistent bone marrow edema in the adjacent bone is of indeterminate significance and may warrant close follow-up. Fluid signal between the repair tissue and subchondral bone indicates delamination, which most commonly occurs during the first 6 months after the procedure. The presence of subchondral cysts beneath the interface also indicates treatment failure[19,20] (**Fig. 16**).

Autologous chondrocyte implantation can be performed in the hip joint but requires surgical hip dislocation, which carries a potential risk of avascular necrosis. Matrix-assisted ACI can be performed in the hip without surgical hip dislocation, and demonstrates promising results.

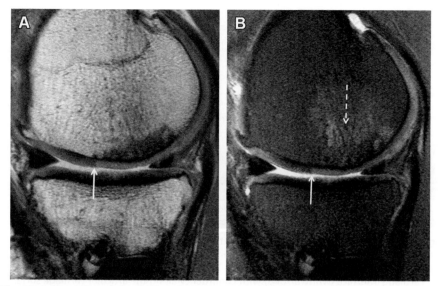

Fig. 13. Sagittal PD-weighted (*A*) and PD FS-weighted (*B*) images demonstrate a high tibial osteotomy and medial femoral condyle OAT system (OATS) with congruency of the graft and native cartilage without an associated fissure (*white arrow*). There is minimal edema in the underlying marrow (*dashed arrow*). The graft was evaluated arthroscopically and appeared intact.

COMPOSITIONAL EVALUATION OF CARTILAGE, AND NEWER IMAGING TECHNIQUES

Newer imaging techniques have been developed that rely on the biology of cartilage to generate images. Although many of these imaging techniques have shown early promise, their use remains primarily experimental with limited clinical applications. Hyaline cartilage consists of 5 layers: the superficial zone, transitional zone, deep zone, tidemark, and the subchondral bone. The cartilage is made up of extracellular matrix

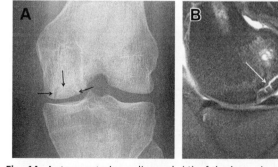
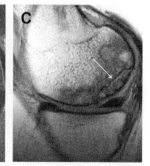

Fig. 14. Anteroposterior radiograph (*A*) of the knee demonstrates a medial femoral condyle osteochondral lesion with a lucent rim surrounding the lesion (*black arrows*). Sagittal PD FS-weighted (*B*) and PD-weighted (*C*) images of the medial femoral condyle in a 23-year-old woman with lupus demonstrates an osteochondral allograft with fluid signal undercutting the graft (*white arrow*) and surrounding marrow edema/sclerosis consistent with graft failure. Additional bone infarcts are incidentally noted related to the underlying lupus.

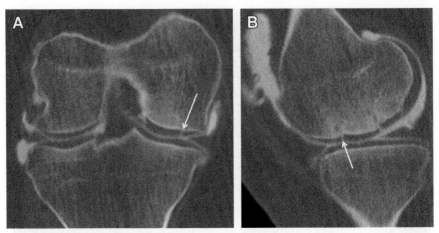

Fig. 15. Coronal (*A*) and sagittal (*B*) reformatted CT arthrogram images obtained after the intra-articular administration of contrast demonstrates a 2-part mosaic-type OATS in the medial condyle performed 10 months prior. There is a persistent cleft at the margins of the cartilage interface (*white arrows*) with congruency along the articular cartilage surface.

(ECM) and chondrocytes. The ECM consists of water, type II collagen, and proteoglycans. Compositional MR imaging techniques specifically target these extracellular molecules and can be differentiated by whether the proteoglycan or collagen component of the ECM is being evaluated. The proteoglycans have GAG side chains with negatively charged carboxylate and sulfate groups. As a result, mobile positively charged sodium ions, or negatively charged gadopentetate dimeglumine ions distribute relative to the proteoglycan concentration. The collagen fibers have an ordered structure and therefore the water associated with them exhibits particular

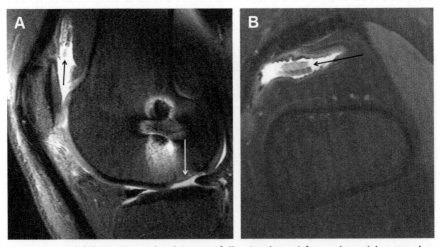

Fig. 16. Sagittal (*A*) PD FS-weighted images following lateral femoral condyle osteochondral cartiform allograft. There is a full-thickness defect involving the lateral femoral condyle consistent with a displaced graft (*white arrow*). A loose body is present in the suprapatellar recess that is confirmed on an axial image (*B*) to be the displaced graft (*black arrow*).

imaging characteristics.[33] The former category includes dGEMRIC, T1 Rho, and sodium MRI, and the latter includes T2 mapping. The goal of these imaging techniques is to theoretically identify cartilage damage before morphologic changes.

Delayed Gadolinium-Enhanced MRI of Cartilage

dGEMRIC imaging is performed after intravenous injection of gadolinium followed by exercising the joint of interest for approximately 10 minutes; 90 minutes after the injection, MRI of the joint of interest is performed. This delay is necessary to allow the gadolinium to penetrate through the full cartilage thickness. The technique relies on the increased accumulation of negatively charged gadolinium salts in injured or degenerated cartilage due to a loss/degradation of the intrinsically negative proteoglycans. A color map is generated based on T1 values within the cartilage, which will vary based on the concentration of gadolinium (**Fig. 17**).

dGEMRIC has been validated in clinical studies in which it was compared against the reference standards of histologic evaluation and quantitative measurements of glycosaminoglycan content within cartilage.[34] It also has been shown to be effective for follow-up in patients who have undergone cartilage repair surgery and regenerative cartilage treatments.[35] The main drawbacks of this imaging technique include the need for intravenous contrast administration and the time required to complete the examination because of the delay between contrast injection and imaging.

Sodium MRI

Sodium MRI relies on signal received directly from sodium ions, rather than hydrogen ions, which are used traditionally for image generation in MRI. There is an abundance of positively charged sodium ions in healthy cartilage that maintain electrical neutrality with the abundant negative charges related to glycosaminoglycans. The density of sodium ions is significantly higher in cartilage compared with the surrounding synovial fluid and bone. Therefore, there will be relatively decreased sodium ion concentration

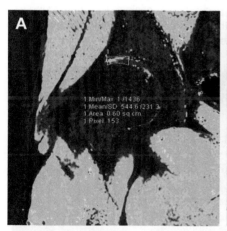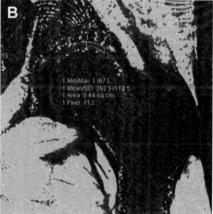

Fig. 17. Coronal dGEMRIC image of the hip with a region of interest drawn through the weight-bearing cartilage demonstrating a mean value of 545 (*A*). This was confirmed to be normal intact cartilage during arthroscopy. Coronal dGEMRIC image of the hip in a different patient with a region of interest drawn through the weight-bearing cartilage demonstrating a mean value of 392 (*B*). Arthroscopy demonstrated grade II chondromalacia involving the acetabular cartilage that was occult on the grayscale MR image.

in areas of diseased cartilage and diminished proteoglycan concentration.[36–38] Sodium MRI requires special hardware, and clinical implementation is difficult, limiting its availability. Studies regarding sodium MRI have shown statistically significant lower sodium MRI values in matrix-associated autologous chondrocyte transplantation.[39] The implication is that the stimulated repair tissue has decreased GAGs, and is less well-equipped to handle compressive loads. An additional study comparing sodium MRI values in patients undergoing bone marrow stimulation through Pridie drilling and microfacture compared with matrix-associated autologous chondrocyte transplantation (MACT) found decreased sodium values in the repaired cartilage compared with native cartilage in both groups. Values were significantly lower in the microfracture group, despite no significant difference in morphologic evaluation of the repair tissue based on the MOCART scoring system.[40] These findings suggest a higher glycosaminoglycan content in the MACT group compared with the microfracture group. One problem with sodium MRI is the relative dearth of sodium ions compared with hydrogen ions of traditional MRI, which decreased overall signal and severely impairs image quality.

T2 Mapping

At its core, MRI is based on the excitation of water molecules in tissue and relaxation back to their equilibrium state. T2 mapping is a measure of the relaxation time of the water within cartilage and is a function of the water content and collagen ultrastructure (**Fig. 18**). This technique generates a color or grayscale map representing the relaxation time for the imaged cartilage. This technique does not require contrast administration, but does require a commercially available software package. Studies have shown that focal increases and heterogeneity of T2 relaxation times within cartilage have been associated with matrix damage and osteoarthritic cartilage.[41] Studies also have shown an increase in T2 relaxation times with age, particularly in the transitional zone of cartilage.[42] There is an improved sensitivity in the detection of cartilage lesions within the knee joint when adding T2 mapping to the routine knee MRI protocol, particularly in the identification of early cartilage lesions.[43] This increased sensitivity is offset by increased imaging and technologist reprocessing time. Although T2 values can identify diseased cartilage, there is no evidence of a linear relationship between T2 values and osteoarthritis grade.[44]

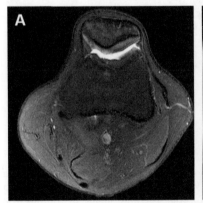 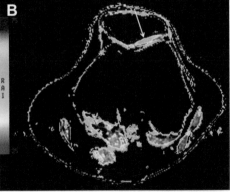

Fig. 18. Axial PD FS-weighted image (*A*) with the corresponding color T2 map (*B*) demonstrates increased T2 mapping signal in the lateral patellar facet (*arrow*) without obvious cartilage injury on the grayscale imaging.

T1 Rho Mapping

T1 rho mapping is a similar imaging technique to T2 mapping in that it is related to the energy generated by spinning protons in relation to their environment. In cartilage tissue, the ECM provides a motion-restricted environment for water molecules. Therefore, changes to the ECM, such as what is seen in proteoglycan depletion, will alter the T1 rho values in the cartilage.[45] In osteoarthritis, damaged hyaline cartilage will have higher T1 rho values than normal cartilage.[46] T1 rho values also may be affected by factors other than proteoglycan depletion and therefore may be less specific than other imaging techniques.[47]

SUMMARY

Articular cartilage lesions represent a growing class of injuries that can be accurately evaluated with MRI. A variety of cartilage repair techniques can be used to potentially treat these lesions. Although functional outcomes remain the primary measure of success, MRI can provide a morphologic and compositional evaluation of the postsurgical cartilage repairs and provide information regarding the progression of these lesions.

REFERENCES

1. McAdams TR, Mithoefer K, Scopp JM, et al. Articular cartilage injury in athletes. Cartilage 2010;1:165–79.
2. Kijowski R, Blankenbaker DG, Davis KW, et al. Comparison of 1.5 and 3.0 T MR imaging for evaluating the articular cartilage of the knee joint. Radiology 2009; 250:839–48.
3. Woertler K, Strothmann M, Tombach B, et al. Detection of articular cartilage lesions: experimental evaluation of low- and high-field-strength MR imaging at 0.18 and 1.0 T. J Magn Reson Imaging 2000;11:678–85.
4. Crema MD, Roemer FW, Zhu Y, et al. Subchondral cystlike lesions develop longitudinally in areas of bone marrow edema-like lesions in patients with or at risk for knee osteoarthritis: detection with MR imaging—the MOST study. Radiology 2010;256:855–62.
5. Rodrigues MB, Camanho GL. MRI evaluation of knee cartilage. Rev Bras Ortop 2010;45:340–6.
6. Crema MD, Roemer FW, Marra MD, et al. Articular cartilage in the knee: current MR imaging techniques and applications in clinical practice and research. Radiographics 2011;31:37–61.
7. Von Engelhardt LV, Lahner M, Kulssmann A, et al. Arthroscopy vs. MRI for a detailed assessment of cartilage disease in osteoarthritis: diagnostic value of MRI in clinical practice. BMC Musculoskelet Disord 2010;11:75.
8. Peterfy CG, Schneider E, Nevitt M. The osteoarthritis initiative: report on the design rationale for the magnetic resonance imaging protocol for the knee. Osteoarthritis Cartilage 2008;16:1433–41.
9. Gold GE, Fuller SE, Hargreaves BA, et al. Driven equilibrium magnetic resonance imaging of articular cartilage: initial clinical experience. J Magn Reson Imaging 2005;21:476–81.
10. Smith TO, Simpson M, Ejindu V, et al. The diagnostic test accuracy of magnetic resonance imaging, magnetic resonance arthrography and computer tomography in the detection of chondral lesions of the hip. Eur J Orthop Surg Traumatol 2013;23:335–44.

11. Van Bergen CJA, Van Den Ende KIM, Brinke BT, et al. Osteochondritis dissecans of the capitellum in adolescents. World J Orthop 2016;7:102–8.

12. Kijowski R, De Smet AA. MRI findings of osteochondritis dissecans of the capitellum with surgical correlation. Am J Roentgenol 2005;185:1453–9.

13. Churchill RW, Munoz J, Ahmad CS. Osteochondritis dissecans of the elbow. Curr Rev Musculoskelet Med 2016;9:232–9.

14. Takahara M, Mura N, Sasaki J, et al. Classification, treatment, and outcome of osteochondritis dissecans of the humeral capitellum. J Bone Joint Surg Am 2007; 89:1205–14.

15. Iannotti JP, Naranja RJJ, Warner JJ. Surgical management of shoulder arthritis in the young and active patient. In: Warner JJ, Iannotti JP, Gerber C, editors. Complex and revision problems in shoulder surgery. Philadelphia: Lippincott-Raven; 1997. p. 289–302.

16. Mccarty LP III, Cole BJ. Nonarthroplasty treatment of glenhumeral cartilage lesions. Arthroscopy 2005;21:1131–42.

17. Beck M, Leunig M, Parvizi J, et al. Anterior femoroacetabular impingement: part II. Midterm results of surgical treatment. Clin Orthop Relat Res 2004;(418):67–73.

18. Ranawat AS, Kelly BT. Function of the labrum and management of labral pathology. Oper Tech Orthopedics 2005;15:239–46.

19. Choi YS, Potter HG, Chun TJ. MR imaging of cartilage repair in the knee and ankle. Radiographics 2008;28:1043–59.

20. Trattnig S, Winalski CS, Marlovits S, et al. Magnetic resonance imaging of cartilage repair: a review. Cartilage 2011;2:5–26.

21. Makris EA, Gomoll AH, Malizos KN, et al. Repair and tissue engineering techniques for articular cartilage. Nat Rev Rheumatol 2015;11:21–34.

22. Potter HG, Foo LF. Magnetic resonance imaging of articular cartilage: trauma, degeneration, and repair. Am J Sports Med 2006;34:661–77.

23. Trattnig S, Millington SA, Szomolanyi P, et al. MR imaging of osteochondral grafts and autologous chondrocyte implantation. Eur Radiol 2007;17:103–18.

24. Kreuz PC, Steinwachs MR, Erggelet C, et al. Results after microfracture of full-thickness chondral defects in different compartments in the knee. Osteoarthritis Cartilage 2006;14(11):1119–25.

25. Mithoefer K, Venugopal V, Manaqibwala M. Incidence, degree, and clinical effect of subchondral bone overgrowth after microfractrue in the knee. Am J Sports Med 2016;44:2057–63.

26. Alparslan L, Winalski CS, Boutin RD, et al. Postoperative magnetic resonance imaging articular cartilage repair. Semin Musculoskelet Radiol 2001;5:345–63.

27. Link TM, Mishung J, Wortler K, et al. Normal and pathological MR findings in osteochondral autografts with longitudinal follow-up. Eur Radiol 2006;16:88–96.

28. Bakay A, Csonge L, Papp G, et al. Osteochondral resurfacing of the knee joint with allograft. Int Orthop 1998;22:277–81.

29. Chahal J, Gross AE, Gross C, et al. Outcomes of osteochondral allograft transplantation. Arthroscopy 2013;29:575–88.

30. Saris D, Price A, Widuchowski W, et al. Matrix-applied characterized autologous cultured chondrocytes versus microfracture: two-year follow-up of a prospective randomized trial. Am J Sports Med 2014;42:1384–94.

31. Peterfy CG, Guermazi A, Zaim S, et al. Whole-organ magnetic resonance imaging score (WORMS) of the knee in osteoarthritis. Osteoarthritis Cartilage 2004;12: 177–90.

32. Marlovits S, Striessnig G, Resinger CT, et al. Definition of pertinent parameters for the evaluation of articular cartilage repair tissue with high-resolution magnetic resonance imaging. Eur J Radiol 2004;52:310–9.
33. Gold GE, Chen CA, Koo S, et al. Recent advances in MRI of articular cartilage. Am J Roentgenol 2009;193:628–38.
34. Bashir A, Gray ML, Hartke J, et al. Nondestructive imaging of human cartilage glycosaminoglycan concentration by MRI. Magn Reson Med 1999;41:857–65.
35. Bekkers JEJ, Bartels LW, Benink RJ, et al. Delayed gadolinium enhanced MRI of cartilage (dGEMRIC) can be effectively applied for longitudinal cohort evaluation of articular cartilage regeneration. Osteoarthritis Cartilage 2013;21:943–9.
36. Borthakur A, Shapiro EM, Beers J, et al. Sensitivity of MRI to proteoglycan depletion in cartilage: comparison of sodium and proton MRI. Osteoarthritis Cartilage 2000;8:288–93.
37. Wang L, Wu Y, Chang G, et al. Rapid isotropic 3D-sodium MRI of the knee joint in vivo at 7T. J Magn Reson Imaging 2009;30:606–14.
38. Wheaton AJ, Borthakur A, Shapiro EM, et al. Proteoglycan loss in human knee cartilage: quantitation with sodium MR imaging—feasibility study. Radiology 2004;231:900–5.
39. Trattnig S, Welsch GH, Juras V, et al. 23Na MR imaging at 7 T after knee matrix-associated autologous chondrocyte transplantation preliminary results. Radiology 2010;257:175–84.
40. Zbyn S, Stelzeneder D, Welsch GH, et al. Evaluation of native hyaline cartilage and repair tissue after two cartilage repair surgery techniques with 23Na MR imaging at 7 T: initial experience. Osteoarthritis Cartilage 2012;20:837–45.
41. Dunn TC, Lu Y, Jin H, et al. T2 relaxation time of cartilage at MR imaging: comparison with severity of knee osteoarthritis. Radiology 2004;232:592–8.
42. Mosher TJ, Dardzinski BJ, Smith MB. Human articular cartilage: influence of aging and early symptomatic degeneration on the spatial variation of T2-preliminary findings at 3T. Radiology 2000;214:259–66.
43. Kijowski R, Blankenbaker DG, Munoz Del Rio A, et al. Evaluation of the articular cartilage of the knee joint: value of adding a T2 mapping sequence to the routine MR imaging protocol. Radiology 2013;267:503–13.
44. Koff MF, Amrami KK, Kaufman KR. Clinical evaluation of T2 values of patellar cartilage in patients with osteoarthritis. Osteoarthritis Cartilage 2007;15:198–204.
45. Duvvuri U, Charagundla SR, Kudchodkar SB, et al. Human knee: in vivo T1(rho)-weighted MR imaging at 1.5 T—preliminary experience. Radiology 2001;220: 822–6.
46. Stahl R, Luke A, Li X, et al. T1 rho, T2 and focal knee cartilage abnormalities in physically active and sedentary healthy subjects versus early OA patients: a 3.0-Tesla MRI study. Eur Radiol 2009;19:132–43.
47. Mlynarik V, Trattnig S, Huber M, et al. The role of relaxation times in monitoring proteoglycan depletion in articular cartilage. J Magn Reson Imaging 1999; 10(4):497–502.

Nonoperative Options for Management of Articular Cartilage Disease

Sourav K. Poddar, MD[a,b,*], Luke Widstrom, DO[a]

KEYWORDS

- Viscosupplementation • Cartilage • Osteoarthritis • Corticosteroid • Glucosamine
- NSAIDs

KEY POINTS

- Low-impact exercise and weight loss are beneficial for osteoarthritis of weight-bearing joints.
- Judicious use of nonsteroidal anti-inflammatory drugs (NSAIDs) and acetaminophen can be appropriate for pain management.
- Topical NSAIDs may be a treatment option with fewer side effects than their oral counterpart.
- Viscosupplementation injections are useful for mild to moderate knee osteoarthritis.
- Corticosteroid injections are useful for short-term pain relief.

INTRODUCTION

Articular cartilage damage is a major cause of pain and functional disability which can occur as a result of injury, disease process such as osteoarthritis, or both. While surgical approaches may provide definitive treatment, they are not typically indicated for mild to moderate damage, may be contraindicated in patients with risk factor, and carry a risk of both operative and anesthetic complications. Nonoperative care may not be definitive in advanced cases, however it can provided definitive treatment in more mild to moderate disease. When excluding biologic options, nonoperative treatments do not reverse the disease process or damage, however there are a variety of options which have been shown to provide significant improvement in terms of pain and function, and many treatments delay and can potentially stall progression of articular cartilage damage. In this chapter, we provide an evidence based approach to the various nonoperative options for the treatment of articular cartilage disease, including

Disclosure Statement: The authors have nothing to disclose.
[a] Department of Family Medicine, University of Colorado School of Medicine, Aurora, CO, USA;
[b] Department of Orthopedics, University of Colorado School of Medicine, Aurora, CO, USA
* Corresponding author. CU Sports Medicine Center, 2000 South Colorado Boulevard, Tower One, Suite 4500, Denver, CO 80222.
E-mail address: sourav.poddar@ucdenver.edu

Clin Sports Med 36 (2017) 447–456
http://dx.doi.org/10.1016/j.csm.2017.02.003
0278-5919/17/© 2017 Elsevier Inc. All rights reserved.

exercise, weight loss, physical therapy, braces, oral medications, topical medications, supplements, corticosteroid injections, viscosupplementation, and prolotherapy.

Exercise

Among nonpharmacologic treatments of osteoarthritis (OA), exercise is one of the most consistently recommended modalities in national and international guidelines. Exercise has been shown to decrease symptoms of OA, improve joint function, and prevent disability.[1] Modalities that are recommended include both land-based and water-based training, as well as strength, flexibility, and endurance training. The Osteoarthritis Research Society International has made recommendations in favor of land-based exercise, water-based exercise, and strength training, all based on good-quality evidence taken from systematic reviews and meta-analyses of randomized controlled trials (RCTs).[2]

A 2015 systematic review of 54 RCTs assessed the immediate and short-term effects of exercise on knee OA.[3] High-quality evidence demonstrated a mean 12-point reduction in pain on a 0 to 100 scale immediately following exercise. Additionally, exercise improved function by an equivalent of 10 points. Twelve studies included in the review analyzed the sustainability of treatment effect after cessation of formal treatment for both pain and physical function over a 2-month to 6-month period. An equivalent reduction of 6 points on the pain scale and improvement of 3 points on the function scale were noted.

A similar systematic review published in 2014 analyzed 10 RCTs pertaining to the treatment benefits of land-based exercise for hip OA.[4] Although not as marked as the effect for knee OA, a significant improvement in both pain and physical function was noted. Pain was reduced by 8 points with exercise, and physical function was improved by 7 points. These improvements were both sustained for 3 to 6 months after the cessation of treatment in the 5 studies that followed patients for this duration.

Thirteen RCTs were included in the most recent systematic review assessing the benefits of aquatic based therapy for both knee and hip OA.[5] Twelve of the studies showed a significant decrease in pain scores by a mean of 5 points and an improvement in disability by a mean of 5 points. Ten of the studies additionally found a mean 7-point higher score on quality of life compared with the control group.

Weight Loss

As a person's weight increases, there is an associated increase in joint pain symptoms and severity.[6] In addition, there is an elevated risk of developing OA with weight gain, up to 36% for every 5 kg. Weight gain can also accelerate the progression of OA and lead to greater severity of disease. This has been demonstrated in cadaveric studies.

However, weight loss has been shown to decrease physical disability due to OA, and meta-analysis has shown that this effect can be predictably reproduced with only a 5% weight reduction over a 20-week period.[7] In addition, pain has been demonstrated to be reduced with weight loss, although a dose-response relationship has not been established. When weight loss is maintained, the benefits of pain reduction continue to be significant, and this has been shown to be true when assessed over a year after initial weight reduction.[8] The improvement in pain and function associated with weight loss may be partially due to a significant reduction in joint compressive forces and inflammatory cytokines.[9] For example, every decrease in 1 kg of weight leads to a 2.2 kg decrease in peak knee load.[10] Notably, this is independent of the effects of exercise, as weight loss due to diet has been shown to have a greater reduction in the aforementioned measures when compared with weight loss due to exercise.[9] Interestingly, this decrease in joint loads and proinflammatory cytokines is seen with increased walking speed. Weight loss has also demonstrated reduced rates of articular cartilage thickness loss and improved articular cartilage quality (as measured by proteoglycan content)[11] in medial compartment knee OA. This has been measured with as little as a 7% reduction in body weight.

The significant benefits of weight loss when measured against the low risks associated have led to strong recommendations in favor of weight loss for overweight persons with OA from multiple organizations including the Osteoarthritis Research Society International (OARSI) and American College of Rheumatology (ACR).[1]

Physical Therapy/Strength Training

One of the most commonly prescribed treatments for articular cartilage disease is physical therapy. Physical therapy includes many methods and modalities, but the component that has the highest level of evidence is strength training. Strength training is one of the core treatments deemed appropriate for all individuals in the OARSI guidelines for nonsurgical management of knee OA.[2] Improved strength can lead to decreased joint loading and increased joint stability.[12] A 2011 systematic review on the effect of strength training for knee OA showed moderate effect size for both decreasing pain and improving function.[2]

Few studies evaluate the effectiveness of physical therapy for delaying progression of OA to the endpoint of joint replacement. A recent RCT of 109 participants with 6-year follow-up compared rates of hip replacement for patients with OA who performed a strengthening, flexibility, and functional exercise program to those who had education alone.[13] At 6 years, survival of the native hip was 44% in the treatment group compared with 25% in the control group, and the mean time to joint replacement was 5.4 years compared with 3.5 years.

Results for investigations evaluating other modalities used in physical therapy, such as transcutaneous electrical nerve stimulation units and therapeutic ultrasound range from showing no benefit to mixed evidence in low-quality studies, and as such these modalities are not recommended.[2,14]

Bracing

Various braces and other biomechanical interventions, such as compression sleeves, foot orthoses, and canes, are used by patients with articular cartilage disease to provide additional structural support in attempts to alleviate pain and improve function. Unloader braces in particular may be used in the knee when either the lateral or medial compartment is predominantly involved in an attempt to offload the affected compartment and distribute forces more evenly. Although in some instances this can make a significant difference, there may be drawbacks to use as unloader braces can be uncomfortable, fit poorly, and limit higher level activities. The evidence for biomechanical interventions overall is inconclusive for benefits in the realms of pain, function, stiffness, and quality of life.[15] There is a lack of agreement among the various major guidelines for the use of these assistive devices for OA.[1] However, as these are low risk interventions, they may be worth a trial with shared decision making. The OARSI recommends the use of biomechanical interventions for knee OA as directed by an appropriate specialist.[2] However, cane use is not recommended for patients with multiple joint involvement as it may increase the weight-bearing load on other affected joints to alleviate knee pain.

ORAL MEDICATIONS: ACETAMINOPHEN, NONSTEROIDAL ANTI-INFLAMMATORY DRUGS, OPIOIDS

When patients are no longer experiencing sufficient symptom relief from nonpharmacologic methods, either oral or topical analgesics are typically initiated as an adjunctive therapy. A logical first choice is acetaminophen due to greater safety and a lower side-effect profile than nonsteroidal anti-inflammatory drugs (NSAIDs). As such, it is consistently recommended as a first-line pharmacologic treatment option.[1] There is low-level evidence on the effectiveness of acetaminophen for OA pain in the short term.[2] A conservative dosing regimen for pain relief as needed and with activity is typically recommended with a maximum dose limited to 3 g a day.

For patients with inflammatory OA, or for those with an inadequate response to acetaminophen, oral NSAIDs can be used either in place of or as an adjunct to acetaminophen. Evidence suggests that NSAIDs are more effective for moderate to severe OA in terms of pain reduction and improvement in functional status.[16] However, this needs to be weighed against the increased risk of gastrointestinal and renal side effects. Gastrointestinal effects may be mitigated by using the cyclo-oxygenase-2 selective inhibitor celecoxib, which has a similar rate to acetaminophen.[17] The rate of cardiac and vascular side effects for celecoxib is higher than placebo, but similar to most nonselective NSAIDs other than naproxen, which has the lowest risk.[18] However, celecoxib, as opposed to the nonselective NSAIDs, has not been demonstrated to have a significantly greater treatment effect than acetaminophen.[17] When considering the gastrointestinal risks of NSAID, providers may contemplate concomitantly initiating a proton pump inhibitor for gastroprotection in patients with moderate comorbidity risk. This has been shown to reduce the rate of endoscopically detected gastroduodenal ulcers.[2] Oral NSAIDs are generally not recommended for patients with high comorbidity risk.

Opioid pain medication is sometimes used for patients with pain from articular cartilage disease that is refractory to acetaminophen, NSAIDs, and injections. However, a 2014 Cochrane review of opioids for knee and hip OA found only a 0.7-cm difference between opioids and placebo on a 0 to 10-cm visual analog pain scale.[19] The difference for function was only 0.6 units on the 0 to 10 WOMAC disability scale. This questionable clinical relevance is contrasted by a significant risk of withdrawal and serious adverse events. As a result, opioids are typically reserved only for patients who have failed all other nonoperative treatments and who are not surgical candidates. In such instances, opioids should be provided under the close observation of a primary care provider, low-potency opioids should be used, and dose escalation should be avoided.

TOPICALS: NONSTEROIDAL ANTI-INFLAMMATORY DRUGS, LIDOCAINE, CAPSAICIN

Another option for patients who want to try pharmacologic treatment but wish to minimize systemic effects is topical therapy. Topical treatments deliver local analgesic effects with minimal systemic absorption. Options include topical NSAIDs, such as diclofenac, lidocaine, and capsaicin. A 2016 Cochrane review evaluated 33 RCTs on topical NSAIDs for chronic musculoskeletal pain due to OA.[20] In studies ranging 6 to 12 weeks, 60% of patients had a significant decrease in pain compared with placebo carrier. However, 50% of patients had similar results with the placebo carrier, showing only a 10% increase in success rate with topical compared with placebo. There was a slight increase in local skin reactions with topical NSAIDs but no increase in gastrointestinal adverse effects compared with placebo. The OARSI recommends topical NSAIDs for patients with knee-only OA but is uncertain for multiple joint involvement.[2]

Capsaicin is the active ingredient in hot chili pepper. When applied locally, it enhances the release of substance P from pain nerve fibers, such that it is rapidly depleted and decreases pain signal transmission.[21] Good evidence has demonstrated that it is superior to placebo for pain reduction, but at the increased risk of local irritation, with up to fourfold number of patients withdrawing from trials due to this.[2] Drug residue on the hands can lead to mucous membrane, eye, and skin irritation in other areas if care is not taken during application.

SUPPLEMENTS: GLUCOSAMINE, CHONDROITIN, OTHERS

Many patients with articular cartilage disease wishing to avoid traditional pharmacologic treatments or their associated side effects turn to over-the-counter supplements. Two of the most commonly used supplements are glucosamine and chondroitin sulfate, either alone or in combination. The estimated $810 million US consumer market for the 2 supplements in 2005 demonstrates the extent of use.[22] The rationale behind glucosamine use is related to its presence in human articular cartilage. Glucosamine is an aminosaccharide used for the synthesis of glycosaminoglycans and glycoproteins, and is highly concentrated in connective tissues, especially cartilage. Chondroitin is a glycosaminoglycan found in the extracellular matrix of articular cartilage.[23] In vitro studies demonstrate that it increases type II collagen and proteoglycan synthesis in human articular chondrocytes, reduce inflammation, and improve the anabolic/catabolic balance of the extracellular matrix.[24]

Despite the prevalence of glucosamine and chondroitin in human articular cartilage and the promising in vitro effects, studies analyzing pain and disease progression have had mixed results. A 2005 systematic review of 25 RCTs comparing glucosamine with placebo for OA found no difference in pain improvement when only considering the high-quality studies, but did show a 22% improvement when including all studies.[25] The same review found statistical improvements in function in the glucosamine group using the Lequesne index but not the WOMAC index. There was no statistical difference from placebo in terms of adverse reactions. A recent meta-analysis evaluated the effectiveness of glucosamine and chondroitin sulfate for chondroprotection. Two of 3 trials used glucosamine sulfate, and both of those trials found a decreased loss of joint space on radiographs and decreased odds of experiencing OA progression compared with placebo.[26] This is in agreement with prior meta-analyses that found small to moderate protective effects on joint space narrowing at 3 years.[27] This was not found to be the case in the trial using glucosamine hydrochlorate.[26]

A 2015 Cochrane review analyzing the effect of chondroitin for OA found improved pain scores compared with placebo but with high heterogeneity and low level evidence.[28] Small but statistically significant improvement in function was demonstrated, as was a decreased loss of joint space compared with placebo. Additionally, the number of adverse events was statistically similar to placebo. A recent double-blinded RCT demonstrated statistically significant reduction in cartilage volume loss in knee medial compartment OA at 2 years compared with celecoxib.[29]

Patients who are interested in taking supplements should be counseled that glucosamine and chondroitin may be beneficial for pain and function, but the effect may be small and the evidence is of low quality. The evidence for chondroprotection for both supplements is of moderate to high quality. Glucosamine sulfate has better evidence than glucosamine hydrochlorate for this purpose. Given these findings and the low risk, both supplements may be worth a trial, but the benefits may take months to years to be realized.

Fish oil is another supplement commonly used by patients with OA. Fish oil is a source of omega-3 fatty acids and has anti-inflammatory properties.[30] The benefits of fish oil for the treatment of rheumatoid arthritis (RA) are well accepted and it has been shown to reduce pain scores and the use of other medications. Due to its efficacy in RA, it has been extrapolated that fish oil may have benefit in OA, especially with its anti-inflammatory function. Most studies, however, have either been in vitro, showing reduced inflammatory cartilage destruction, or in vivo animal studies, with an example being noticeable improvement of signs of pain in dogs. Few human RCTs have been performed. A 2015 meta-analysis found only 6 such studies since 1992, with significantly varying endpoints and methods of evaluation and predominantly low quality.[30] The results were mixed with some studies showing no benefit, some showing modest benefit, and some showing significant benefit. More high-quality studies are needed in this area before any recommendations can be made.

STEROID INJECTIONS

Although it has been described as a degenerative process, current understanding of the pathophysiology of OA involves a cascade of inflammatory mediators in the joint. Corticosteroid injections are performed with the intention of reducing pain and improving function by producing a powerful local anti-inflammatory effect.[31] The effects of corticosteroid injections are most notable in the short term, resulting in significant decreases in pain.[2] This makes steroid injections a reasonable option for acute flares of OA or other causes of acute onset pain due to articular cartilage insult. The benefits after 1 to 6 weeks, however, are unclear.[31] Hyaluronic acid injections have greater evidence for longer duration relief.[32] However, from a practical clinical standpoint, many insurance companies require failure of corticosteroid injections before a trial of viscosupplementation. This often results in the use of a trial of corticosteroid injections for OA even if long-term relief from chronic pain is the desired effect.

There is a paucity of data comparing the efficacy of the various corticosteroids. The presence of only a small number of high-quality RCTs and mixed results prevents the establishment of firm conclusions to guide treatment.[33]

The most common side effects of corticosteroid injection are injection site pain, elevated blood sugar, and rarely skin atrophy.[33] However, a Cochrane review indicated that placebo injections resulted in higher rates of side effects than corticosteroids.[31] The rate of joint infection when using sterile technique has been estimated at approximately 1 in 22,000 injections.[34] There is some concern that steroid injections may accelerate cartilage loss. This may be due to animal studies with rabbits in which frequent administration and high dosages demonstrated this effect. However, other animal studies have had mixed results, and in some instances have shown beneficial effects on cartilage structure.[35] One study comparing triamcinolone acetonide injections to saline injections in the knee every 3 months for 2 years showed no difference in joint space loss.[36]

VISCOSUPPLEMENTATION

Viscosupplementation is a technique that involves the injection of exogenous high molecular weight hyaluronic acid molecules to combat the effect of the decreased viscoelasticity of synovial fluid seen in OA.[37] It is typically the second-line choice for injection therapy if the effectiveness of corticosteroids is limited. It is also used without prior corticosteroid injections for younger, physically active patients. Viscosupplementation is a good alternative in situations in which corticosteroid injections are contraindicated, such as with labile diabetes mellitus, or in the setting of adverse reaction or allergy to steroid preparations. Although pain relief from viscosupplementation is usually slower in onset than corticosteroid injections, it typically confers longer-lasting pain relief, and may be a better intermediate-term option due to its decreased side-effect profile.[32]

In addition to the traditionally understood biomechanical model of viscosupplementation increasing joint lubrication and shock absorption by providing improved visco-elasticity, several other mechanisms for pain reduction are at play. It has been shown to stimulate endogenous production of hyaluronic acid by synovial cells.[37] It may also have an anti-inflammatory effect by blocking production of prostaglandin E2 and release of arachidonic acid. Research suggests it might have a direct analgesic on intra-articular nociceptors. Finally, viscosupplementation may offer a protective effect against cell damage from oxygen free radicals and phagocytosis.[38]

A 2006 Cochrane review of 76 RCTs on viscosupplementation for knee OA concluded that it is an effective treatment with beneficial effects for pain, function, and patient global assessment.[32] This was most notable at the 5-week to 13-week period for pain with weight bearing. When compared with placebo, the effect size at some time points was moderate to large. However, the onset, duration, and magnitude of effect varied between the various products and time points of administration.

In 2016 the American Medical Society for Sports Medicine released a position statement on the use of hyaluronic acid injections for knee OA based on the results of a meta-analysis of literature comparing hyaluronic acid injections to corticosteroid injections and placebo injections.[39] The meta-analysis evaluated studies that determined a significant clinical response based on the Outcome Measures in Rheumatoid Arthritis Clinical Trials-ORSI (OMERACT-OARSI) criteria. They found that compared with steroid and placebo injections, hyaluronic acid injections led to a 15% and 11% higher response rate, respectively. This led to a recommendation in favor of hyaluronic acid injections for appropriate patients with mild to moderate knee OA.

Viscosupplementation for joints other than the knee has less robust evidence, generally with insufficient evidence to make recommendations for or against use.[40] For example, a recent systematic review of hyaluronic acid injections for ankle OA found that although it is safe and effective, it was no more effective than other conservative treatments.[41] Although a recent meeting of 8 European experts on OA led to a unanimous vote in favor of the effectiveness of viscosupplementation for mild to moderate knee OA, there was only moderate consensus in favor for hip and ankle, and weak consensus in favor for shoulder OA.[42] The OARSI deemed hyaluronic acid injections for hip OA as not appropriate.[2]

PROLOTHERAPY (AND BIOLOGICS)

Prolotherapy is an injection technique that uses nonbiologic irritant solutions, most commonly dextrose.[43] The mechanism of action is multifactorial and not well understood, but proposed mechanisms include stimulation of a local healing process in tissue with chronic damage, decreasing joint instability by increasing the strength of tendons and ligaments, and stimulating cell proliferation.[44] Animal studies have suggested cartilage-specific anabolic growth. A recent small study used arthroscopic second look after treatment along with staining for chondrocyte growth and biopsy of sites with increased stain uptake.[43] The biopsies revealed a mixture of fibrocartilage and hyalinelike cartilage.

A recent meta-analysis of 4 RCTs demonstrated that peri-articular and intra-articular hypertonic dextrose prolotherapy is superior to exercise alone for improvement in pain and function in knee OA, meeting criteria for statistically significant and clinically relevant effect, but with moderate heterogeneity.[44] A 2013 RCT with 90 participants compared dextrose prolotherapy with saline injections and exercise for knee OA.[45] At 52 weeks, the prolotherapy arm had a significant improvement over the saline and exercise arms in the 100-point WOMAC composite score, which evaluates knee pain, function, and stiffness. The prolotherapy group had a mean improvement of 15.3 points compared with 7.6 and 8.2 for the saline and exercise groups. Although prolotherapy may be an effective form of treatment for OA, patient discomfort with needle sticks, lack of insurance coverage, and finding a prolotherapist provide treatment challenges.[46]

Other biologic treatment options, such as platelet rich plasma and bone marrow aspirate concentrate/stem cells are also currently used for the treatment of OA. These provide a fertile environment for further study and are covered in detail in the article (see Matthew J. Kraeutler and colleagues' article, "Biologic Options for Articular Cartilage Wear (Platelet-Rich Plasma, Stem Cells, Bone Marrow Aspirate Concentrate)," in this issue).

SUMMARY

Nonoperative options for articular cartilage injury are omnipresent but have not shown to be curative. Recommendations for low-impact exercise and weight loss provide benefit and are a foundation for the treatment of OA. Many options are available to manage the pain associated with OA and their use should be based on an individualized consideration of the risks and benefits afforded the patient. Future studies to individualize treatment options based on patient phenotype and genotype may hold promise.

REFERENCES

1. Nelson AE, Allen KD, Golightly YM, et al. A systematic review of recommendations and guidelines for the management of osteoarthritis: the chronic osteoarthritis management initiative of the U.S. bone and joint initiative. Semin Arthritis Rheum 2014;43(6):701–12.
2. McAlindon TE, Bannuru RR, Sullivan MC, et al. OARSI guidelines for the non-surgical management of knee osteoarthritis. Osteoarthritis Cartilage 2014;22(3): 363–88.
3. Fransen M, McConnell S, Harmer AR, et al. Exercise for osteoarthritis of the knee. Cochrane Database Syst Rev 2015;(1):CD004376.
4. Fransen M, McConnell S, Hernandez-Molina G, et al. Exercise for osteoarthritis of the hip. Cochrane Database Syst Rev 2014;(4):CD007912.
5. Bartels EM, Juhl CB, Christensen R, et al. Aquatic exercise for the treatment of knee and hip osteoarthritis. Cochrane Database Syst Rev 2016;(3):CD005523.
6. Vincent HK, Heywood K, Connelly J, et al. Obesity and weight loss in the treatment and prevention of osteoarthritis. PM R 2012;4(5 Suppl):S59–67.
7. Christensen R, Bartels EM, Astrup A, et al. Effect of weight reduction in obese patients diagnosed with knee osteoarthritis: a systematic review and meta-analysis. Ann Rheum Dis 2007;66(4):433–9.
8. Christensen R, Henriksen M, Leeds AR, et al. Effect of weight maintenance on symptoms of knee osteoarthritis in obese patients: a twelve-month randomized controlled trial. Arthritis Care Res (Hoboken) 2015;67(5):640–50.
9. Messier SP, Mihalko SL, Legault C, et al. Effects of intensive diet and exercise on knee joint loads, inflammation, and clinical outcomes among overweight and obese adults with knee osteoarthritis: the IDEA randomized clinical trial. JAMA 2013;310(12):1263–73.
10. Aaboe J, Bliddal H, Messier SP, et al. Effects of an intensive weight loss program on knee joint loading in obese adults with knee osteoarthritis. Osteoarthritis Cartilage 2011;19(7):822–8.

11. Anandacoomarasamy A, Leibman S, Smith G, et al. Weight loss in obese people has structure-modifying effects on medial but not on lateral knee articular cartilage. Ann Rheum Dis 2012;71(1):26–32.

12. Nguyen C, Lefèvre-Colau MM, Poiraudeau S, et al. Rehabilitation (exercise and strength training) and osteoarthritis: a critical narrative review. Ann Phys Rehabil Med 2016;59(3):190–5.

13. Svege I, Nordsletten L, Fernandes L, et al. Exercise therapy may postpone total hip replacement surgery in patients with hip osteoarthritis: a long-term follow-up of a randomised trial. Ann Rheum Dis 2015;74(1):164–9.

14. Sharma L. Osteoarthritis year in review 2015: clinical. Osteoarthritis Cartilage 2016;24(1):36–48.

15. Duivenvoorden T, Brouwer RW, van Raaij TM, et al. Braces and orthoses for treating osteoarthritis of the knee. Cochrane Database Syst Rev 2015;(3):CD004020.

16. Towheed TE, Maxwell L, Judd MG, et al. Acetaminophen for osteoarthritis. Cochrane Database Syst Rev 2006;(1):CD004257.

17. Bannuru RR, Schmid CH, Kent DM, et al. Comparative effectiveness of pharmacologic interventions for knee osteoarthritis: a systematic review and network meta-analysis. Ann Intern Med 2015;162(1):46–54.

18. Bhala N, Emberson J, Merhi A, et al. Vascular and upper gastrointestinal effects of non-steroidal anti-inflammatory drugs: meta-analyses of individual participant data from randomised trials. Lancet 2013;382(9894):769–79.

19. da Costa BR, Nüesch E, Kasteler R, et al. Oral or transdermal opioids for osteoarthritis of the knee or hip. Cochrane Database Syst Rev 2014;(9):CD003115.

20. Derry S, Conaghan P, Da Silva JA, et al. Topical NSAIDs for chronic musculoskeletal pain in adults. Cochrane Database Syst Rev 2016;(4):CD007400.

21. Rains C, Bryson HM. Topical capsaicin. A review of its pharmacological properties and therapeutic potential in post-herpetic neuralgia, diabetic neuropathy and osteoarthritis. Drugs Aging 1995;7(4):317–28.

22. Dahmer S, Schiller RM. Glucosamine. Am Fam Physician 2008;78(4):471–6.

23. Uebelhart D, Thonar EJ, Delmas PD, et al. Effects of oral chondroitin sulfate on the progression of knee osteoarthritis: a pilot study. Osteoarthritis Cartilage 1998;6(Suppl A):39–46.

24. Hochberg M, Chevalier X, Henrotin Y, et al. Symptom and structure modification in osteoarthritis with pharmaceutical-grade chondroitin sulfate: what's the evidence? Curr Med Res Opin 2013;29(3):259–67.

25. Towheed TE, Maxwell L, Anastassiades TP, et al. Glucosamine therapy for treating osteoarthritis. Cochrane Database Syst Rev 2005;(2):CD002946.

26. Gallagher B, Tjoumakaris FP, Harwood MI, et al. Chondroprotection and the prevention of osteoarthritis progression of the knee: a systematic review of treatment agents. Am J Sports Med 2015;43(3):734–44.

27. Lee YH, Woo JH, Choi SJ, et al. Effect of glucosamine or chondroitin sulfate on the osteoarthritis progression: a meta-analysis. Rheumatol Int 2010;30(3):357–63.

28. Singh JA, Noorbaloochi S, MacDonald R, et al. Chondroitin for osteoarthritis. Cochrane Database Syst Rev 2015;(1):CD005614.

29. Pelletier JP, Raynauld JP, Beaulieu AD, et al. Chondroitin sulfate efficacy versus celecoxib on knee osteoarthritis structural changes using magnetic resonance imaging: a 2-year multicentre exploratory study. Arthritis Res Ther 2016;18(1):256.

30. Boe C, Vangsness CT. Fish oil and osteoarthritis: current evidence. Am J Orthop (Belle Mead NJ) 2015;44(7):302–5.

31. Jüni P, Hari R, Rutjes AW, et al. Intra-articular corticosteroid for knee osteoarthritis. Cochrane Database Syst Rev 2015;(10):CD005328.
32. Bellamy N, Campbell J, Robinson V, et al. Viscosupplementation for the treatment of osteoarthritis of the knee. Cochrane Database Syst Rev 2006;(2):CD005321.
33. Garg N, Perry L, Deodhar A. Intra-articular and soft tissue injections, a systematic review of relative efficacy of various corticosteroids. Clin Rheumatol 2014;33(12): 1695–706.
34. Pal B, Morris J. Perceived risks of joint infection following intra-articular corticosteroid injections: a survey of rheumatologists. Clin Rheumatol 1999;18(3):264–5.
35. Vandeweerd JM, Zhao Y, Nisolle JF, et al. Effect of corticosteroids on articular cartilage: have animal studies said everything? Fundam Clin Pharmacol 2015; 29(5):427–38.
36. Raynauld JP, Buckland-Wright C, Ward R, et al. Safety and efficacy of long-term intraarticular steroid injections in osteoarthritis of the knee: a randomized, double-blind, placebo-controlled trial. Arthritis Rheum 2003;48(2):370–7.
37. Jackson DW, Evans NA, Thomas BM. Accuracy of needle placement into the intra-articular space of the knee. J Bone Joint Surg Am 2002;84-A(9):1522–7.
38. Presti D, Scott JE. Hyaluronan-mediated protective effect against cell damage caused by enzymatically produced hydroxyl (OH.) radicals is dependent on hyaluronan molecular mass. Cell Biochem Funct 1994;12(4):281–8.
39. Trojian TH, Concoff AL, Joy SM, et al. AMSSM scientific statement concerning viscosupplementation injections for knee osteoarthritis: importance for individual patient outcomes. Clin J Sport Med 2016;26(1):1–11.
40. Conrozier T. Optimizing the effectiveness of viscosupplementation in non-knee osteoarthritis. Joint Bone Spine 2016;83(1):1–2.
41. Faleiro TB, Schulz Rda S, Jambeiro JE, et al. Viscosupplementation in ankle osteoarthritis: a systematic review. Acta Ortop Bras 2016;24(1):52–4.
42. Henrotin Y, Raman R, Richette P, et al. Consensus statement on viscosupplementation with hyaluronic acid for the management of osteoarthritis. Semin Arthritis Rheum 2015;45(2):140–9.
43. Reeves KD, Sit RW, Rabago DP. Dextrose prolotherapy: a narrative review of basic science, clinical research, and best treatment recommendations. Phys Med Rehabil Clin N Am 2016;27(4):783–823.
44. Sit RW, Chung VCh, Reeves KD, et al. Hypertonic dextrose injections (prolotherapy) in the treatment of symptomatic knee osteoarthritis: a systematic review and meta-analysis. Sci Rep 2016;6:25247.
45. Rabago D, Patterson JJ, Mundt M, et al. Dextrose prolotherapy for knee osteoarthritis: a randomized controlled trial. Ann Fam Med 2013;11(3):229–37.
46. Slattengren AH, Christensen T, Prasad S, et al. PURLs: prolotherapy: a nontraditional approach to knee osteoarthritis. J Fam Pract 2014;63(4):206–8.

Biologic Options for Articular Cartilage Wear (Platelet-Rich Plasma, Stem Cells, Bone Marrow Aspirate Concentrate)

CrossMark

Matthew J. Kraeutler, MD[a], Jorge Chahla, MD[b],
Robert F. LaPrade, MD, PhD[b], Cecilia Pascual-Garrido, MD[c],*

KEYWORDS

- Articular cartilage • Platelet-rich plasma • Stem cells
- Bone marrow aspirate concentrate

KEY POINTS

- Biological treatments for articular cartilage repair have gained in popularity in the past decade.
- Advantages of these therapies include minimal invasiveness, improved healing time, and faster recovery.
- Biological therapies for cartilage repair include platelet-rich plasma, bone marrow aspirate concentrate, and cell-based therapies.
- These methods have the added benefit of containing growth factors and/or stem cells that aid in recovery and regeneration.
- The purpose of this article was to review the current cartilage treatment options and the existing literature on outcomes, complications, and safety profile of these products for use in the knee and hip joints.

INTRODUCTION

Articular cartilage damage is a serious clinical and economic burden for the orthopedic community and the public health system. The most common forms that affect articular cartilage include focal chondral lesions and early osteoarthritis (OA). Recently, identifying and treating cases of early OA has become an important

[a] Department of Orthopedics, University of Colorado School of Medicine, 1635 Aurora Ct, Aurora, CO 80045, USA; [b] Steadman Philippon Research Institute, 181 West Meadow Drive, Suite 400, Vail, CO 81657, USA; [c] Department of Orthopedics, Washington University, 660 South Euclid Avenue, Campus Box 8233, St Louis, MO 63110, USA
* Corresponding author.
E-mail address: pascualgarridoc@wudosis.wustl.edu

Clin Sports Med 36 (2017) 457–468
http://dx.doi.org/10.1016/j.csm.2017.02.004
0278-5919/17/© 2017 Elsevier Inc. All rights reserved.

concern, because many patients with painful OA already have extensive structural disease that may preclude treatment with nonoperative modalities. Isolated chondral lesions are also a prevalent pathology seen by orthopedic surgeons. These lesions have been reported in up to 57.3% of all patients undergoing knee arthroscopy, with Outerbridge grade 3 or 4 lesions found in 5.2% of all patients with a diagnosed cartilage lesion.[1] In those undergoing knee arthroscopy for meniscal pathology, 32% of patients in their 20s have been shown to have Outerbridge changes to the articular surfaces of the knee joint.[2]

Procedures available for articular cartilage repair are constantly evolving and in recent years, the focus has shifted from surgical procedures to that of biological interventions. Biological therapies provide a less-invasive and less-expensive alternative to surgery, and therefore represent a potential attractive option for patients with articular cartilage lesions or early OA. The purpose of this article was to review the current cartilage treatment options and the existing literature on outcomes, complications, and safety profile of these biologic products for use in the knee and hip joints.

PLATELET-RICH PLASMA

The use of platelet-rich plasma (PRP) has gained significant attention throughout the orthopedic community in recent years.[3] PRP refers to autologous blood that has been centrifuged to produce a higher concentration of platelets than average.[4,5] A number of studies have attempted to determine the optimal concentration of platelets for purposes of musculoskeletal healing.[6–8] Recently, Fleming and colleagues[6] evaluated the effect of PRP supplementation on graft healing following anterior cruciate ligament (ACL) reconstruction in minipigs using either $1 \times$ (n = 10), $3 \times$ (n = 10), or $5 \times$ (n = 10) PRP concentrations. Interestingly, only the $1 \times$ platelet concentration improved healing over traditional ACL reconstruction. Similarly, Yoshida and colleagues[7] found that, after suspending porcine ACL fibroblasts in various platelet concentrations of PRP, $1 \times$ PRP significantly outperformed $5 \times$ PRP in terms of type I and type III collagen gene expression, apoptosis prevention, and cell metabolism stimulation. Weibrich and colleagues[8] found that an intermediate concentration of platelets ($2–6\times$) resulted in optimal peri-implant bone regeneration in rabbits.

Various formulations of PRP exist. In addition to controlling the concentration of platelets, the white blood cell concentration also may be controlled, with leukocyte-rich PRP (LR-PRP) and leukocyte-poor PRP (LP-PRP) both being used in the literature. No randomized or prospective clinical studies have been performed to compare outcomes between LR-PRP versus LP-PRP,[4] although a recent meta-analysis found improved functional outcome scores with LP-PRP for the treatment of knee OA in comparison with hyaluronic acid (HA) and placebo.[9] A number of randomized clinical trials have demonstrated a positive effect of LP-PRP on OA in comparison with placebo[10] or HA.[11,12] On the other hand, 2 randomized clinical trials have demonstrated no significant difference in outcomes between LR-PRP and HA for the treatment of OA.[13,14] Based on these studies, more consistent literature exists regarding LP-PRP for intra-articular usage.

There is some debate as to the effects of PRP at the cellular layer. Although some investigators believe that the effects of PRP are due mainly to its anti-inflammatory effects, rather than changing the progression of OA,[15] there is evidence that it promotes chondrogenic differentiation in vitro and leads to enhanced cartilage repair in animal models.[16]

In a randomized clinical trial of patients with Kellgren-Lawrence (K-L) grade II to IV knee OA undergoing knee arthroscopy, Duif and colleagues[17] reported short-term improvement in patients receiving intra-articular injections of PRP during surgery compared with a control group. Patients in the intervention group demonstrated significantly better visual analog scale (VAS) pain scores ($P = .008$), Lysholm scores ($P = .033$), and SF-36 physical component summary scores ($P = .027$) at 6-month follow-up. However, no difference was found between intervention and control groups at 12-month follow-up in terms of pain and SF-36 scores.

In another randomized clinical trial of 192 patients with unilateral knee OA (K-L grade 0 to III), Filardo and colleagues[13] compared outcomes of 3 weekly intra-articular injections of LR-PRP versus HA. At 12-month follow-up, patients in both groups demonstrated significant improvement compared with pretreatment in terms of the subjective International Knee Documentation Committee (IKDC) and Tegner scores. However, no significant intergroup difference was demonstrated in IKDC, Tegner, Knee Injury and Osteoarthritis Outcome Scores (KOOS), or EuroQol visual analog scale (EQ-VAS) at 2-month, 6-month, or 12-month follow-up.

Fewer studies have investigated the effects of PRP on hip OA, although recently Dallari and colleagues[18] performed a randomized controlled trial on 111 patients to compare the efficacy of autologous PRP, HA, and a combination of both for the treatment of hip OA. Patients and health care providers were not blinded to the treatments used, although the data collectors and analysts were blinded. Patients received 3 intra-articular ultrasound-guided injections 1 week apart during outpatient surgery, although the types of surgical procedures were not mentioned. In addition, the leukocyte concentration of the PRP formulations was not mentioned. Patients were assessed at 2, 6, and 12 months after treatment. The PRP group demonstrated lower VAS pain scores at all follow-up times and significantly better Western Ontario and McMaster Universities Arthritis Index (WOMAC) scores at the 2-month and 6-month follow-up periods.

Battaglia and colleagues[19] also performed a nonblinded, randomized trial comparing ultrasound-guided PRP versus HA injections for hip OA in 100 consecutive patients. Patients underwent 3 injections every 2 weeks of 5 mL autologous PRP or 2 mL HA. The PRP samples were obtained through a double-spin technique to create a sixfold platelet count. Using the Harris Hip Score (HHS) and VAS, patients in both groups demonstrated significant improvements between 1-month and 3-month follow-up. Although patients showed progressive worsening of symptoms between 6-month and 12-month follow-up, scores were still significantly improved compared with baseline ($P<.0005$). No significant differences were found between the PRP and HA groups.

In terms of focal chondral defects, limited studies in animal models have demonstrated successful results with intra-articular injections of PRP[20] and autologous conditioned plasma (ACP)[21] and the use of an autologous platelet-enriched fibrin scaffold,[22] although similar studies have not been published with human subjects. However, PRP has shown promising results in conjunction with the surgical treatment of knee[17] or hip OA[18] or as a nonoperative treatment modality for these pathologies[19] (**Table 1**). Overall, PRP for knee OA has demonstrated short-term improvement in pain and function.[16] As indications for PRP continue to expand, it will become increasingly important for future studies to state specific methodologies used in the preparation of PRP to recognize ideal preparation techniques and the ideal number of PRP injections for each pathology.[4]

Intra-articular PRP injections have shown promising results in the treatment of knee and hip OA at short-term follow-up periods up to 12 months following injection. However, the long-term effects of these treatments are still unknown, and their results in comparison to injections of HA (viscosupplementation) are also undetermined.

Table 1
Clinical studies on biological treatments for knee and hip articular cartilage lesions

Treatment	Study	Indication	Maximum Follow-Up, mo	Outcome Measures
PRP	Filardo et al,[13] 2015	Knee OA	12	IKDC, KOOS, EQ-VAS, Tegner score
	Duif et al,[17] 2015	Knee OA	12	VAS pain, Lysholm score, SF-36
	Dallari et al,[18] 2016	Hip OA	12	HHS, VAS, WOMAC
	Battaglia et al,[19] 2013	Hip OA	12	HHS, VAS
BMAC	Kim et al,[24] 2014	Knee OA	12	VAS pain, IKDC, SF-36, KOOS, Lysholm
	Hauser & Orlofsky,[25] 2013	Hip, knee, or ankle OA	6 wk	Pain, stiffness, range of motion, crepitus, ability to exercise
	Gobbi et al,[27] 2011	Knee chondral lesions	24	VAS, IKDC, KOOS, Lysholm, Marx, SF-36, Tegner
	Gobbi et al,[28] 2016	Knee chondral lesions	48	MRI, KOOS, IKDC, VAS, Tegner
MSCs	Emadedin et al,[42] 2015	Knee, ankle, or hip OA	30	Walking distance, VAS, WOMAC score
	Pers et al,[43] 2016	Knee OA	6	Safety, WOMAC
	Soler et al,[44] 2016	Knee OA	48	VAS, HAQ, SF-36, Lequesne functional index, WOMAC
	Kim et al,[45] 2015	Knee OA	28	IKDC, Tegner score, ICRS grade

Abbreviations: BMAC, bone marrow aspirate concentrate; EQ-VAS, EuroQol visual analog scale; HAQ, health assessment questionnaire; HHS, Harris Hip Score; ICRS, International Cartilage Repair Society; IKDC, International Knee Documentation Committee; KOOS, Knee Injury and Osteoarthritis Outcome Score; MSCs, mesenchymal stem cells; OA, osteoarthritis; PRP, platelet-rich plasma; VAS, visual analog scale; WOMAC, Western Ontario and McMaster Universities Arthritis Index.

Furthermore, the effects of PRP injections on focal chondral defects in human subjects has not been demonstrated.

BONE MARROW ASPIRATE CONCENTRATE

Bone marrow aspirate concentrate (BMAC) has experienced a rise in popularity because it is one of the few US Food and Drug Administration (FDA)-approved methods for delivering stem cells.[23] BMAC is most often formulated from iliac or tibial bone marrow, which is extracted and mixed with anticoagulants and batroxobin enzyme, although other methods of activation have been reported.[23–25] The quality of the bone marrow aspirate can be improved by aspirating at multiple locations with a small syringe. Hernigou and colleagues[26] found that, when aspirating bone marrow from the iliac crest, progenitor cell concentrations were on average 300% higher using a 10-mL syringe compared with a 50-mL syringe (P<.01). The bone marrow extraction procedure typically has minimal interference with daily activities, with 3 hours of bed rest immediately after the procedure and restrictions on extreme exercise for 6 weeks postoperatively.[24] The most commonly reported side effects are joint pain and swelling.[23]

The concentration of stem cells in BMAC is relatively low (0.001% to 0.01% of mononuclear cells following centrifugation). In addition to stem cells, BMAC contains growth factors that may assist in the regeneration and preservation of cartilage, and have been shown to have anti-inflammatory and anabolic effects on the injected tissue (**Table 2**).[23] The growth factors present in BMAC include platelet-derived growth factor, transforming growth factor-beta (TGF-β), and bone morphogenetic protein (BMP)-2 and BMP-7.[23]

In a case series of 41 patients (75 knees) with knee OA (K-L grades I to IV), Kim and colleagues[24] evaluated outcomes of BMAC injection with adipose tissue. At 12-month follow-up, VAS pain score, IKDC, SF-36, KOOS, and Lysholm scores increased among the group compared with preoperative scores, although statistical significance was not mentioned in this study. A significant association was found between higher K-L grade and inferior outcomes at follow-up. Overall, joint swelling (92%) and pain (41%) were the most common side effects experienced by patients.

In a small case series of 7 patients with hip, knee, or ankle OA, Hauser and Orlofsky[25] performed intra-articular injections (mean 4.1 injections per patient) with unfractionated whole bone marrow in combination with hyperosmotic dextrose. At a minimum 6-week follow-up, 5 of 7 patients noted complete relief or strong functional improvement. Based on a VAS from 0 (complete relief) to 10 (maximum limitation), average pain intensity scores improved from 6.2 preoperatively to 0.07 at follow-up ($P = .002$). Likewise, joint stiffness improved from 7.0 to 0.7 ($P = .002$). No adverse events were noted.

In terms of focal chondral defects, Gobbi and colleagues[27] performed a prospective case series of 15 patients with grade IV knee chondral lesions undergoing operative

Table 2 Biological therapy comparison			
Treatment	PRP	BMAC	Stem Cells
Invasiveness	Minimal	Moderate	Moderate
Presence of stem cells	None	Minimal	High
Presence of growth factors	High	High	None

Abbreviations: BMAC, bone marrow aspirate concentrate; PRP, platelet-rich plasma.

transplantation with BMAC covered with a collagen I/III matrix (Chondro-Gide; Geistlich, Wolhusen, Switzerland). The average lesion size was 9.2 cm^2 and 6 of 15 patients had multiple chondral lesions. At a final follow-up of 24 months, patients showed significant improvement (P<.005) in VAS, IKDC, KOOS, Lysholm, Marx, SF-36, and Tegner scores compared with preoperative scores. In 3 patients who underwent a second-look arthroscopy with concomitant biopsy at 2-year follow-up, hyaline-like histologic findings were found for all samples. Furthermore, no adverse events were reported in this study.

Gobbi and colleagues[28] also performed a prospective cohort study in patients with International Cartilage Repair Society (ICRS) grade IV chondral lesions in the knee. Patients were treated operatively with a hyaluronan-based scaffold (Hyalofast; Anika Therapeutics Inc, Bedford, MA) soaked in BMAC. A study group of patients older than 45 years (n = 20) was compared with a control group younger than 45 years (n = 20). At a final follow-up of 4 years, the following outcome scores significantly improved for both groups: all KOOS subscores, Tegner score, and subjective IKDC (all P<.001). Results in the study group were affected by lesion size, with a significantly better subjective IKDC score (P = .006) and a trend toward a significantly better KOOS pain score (P = .086) in patients with lesions smaller than 8 cm^2 compared with larger than 8 cm^2 at final follow-up. Based on MRI, greater than 50% filling of the defect was observed in 81% and 71% of patients in the study and control groups, respectively, at final follow-up. Overall, 2 patients experienced persistent subchondral bone edema, but otherwise no major adverse reactions were reported.

Few studies have reported outcomes of BMAC for knee or hip cartilage defects, although the outcomes in these studies are good to excellent overall.[23] Patients with mild OA and smaller focal chondral defects have been shown to benefit more from BMAC than those with severe OA (as assessed by the K-L scale) and larger defects. As with PRP, long-term outcomes have not yet been reported by multiple studies.

STEM CELLS (CONNECTIVE TISSUE PROGENITORS)

Connective tissue progenitors (CTPs) are defined as proliferative cells capable of differentiating into various connective tissue phenotypes.[29] Thus, the term CTP not only encapsulates pluripotent stem cells but also progenitors derived from stem cells that may be at various stages of cellular commitment.

Stem cells are defined as undifferentiated cells that are capable of proliferation, regeneration, self-maintenance, and replication.[30] Human embryonic stem cells (hESCs), induced pluripotent stem cells (iPSCs), and mesenchymal stem cells (MSCs) have all been used for treatment of OA.[15] Due to their accessibility, MSCs are the most popular stem cell option for articular cartilage repair.[31] Furthermore, it is more difficult to ensure homogeneity in cell division with iPSCs or hESCs than with MSCs.[32] MSCs are present in a range of tissue types, have anti-inflammatory effects, can be harvested in large quantities, and are shown to produce proteins conducive to cartilage regeneration.[33] In 2006, the Mesenchymal and Tissue Stem Cell Committee of the International Society for Cellular Therapy defined the following minimal criteria for a human cell to be classified as an MSC: (1) the ability to adhere to plastic when maintained in standard culture conditions; (2) expression of CD105, CD73, and CD90; (3) lack of expression of CD45, CD34, CD14, or CD11b, CD79alpha, or CD19 and HLA-DR surface molecules; and (4) the ability to differentiate to osteoblasts, adipocytes, and chondroblasts in vitro.[34] Without meeting these criteria, the term MSC should not be used.

Chang and colleagues[31] suggested that MSCs also have anti-inflammatory elements, as preclinical trials in small mammals observed an anti-inflammatory response. Because of their easy accessibility and minimal morbidity caused during harvest, adipose-derived stem cells (ASCs) result in a high yield of stem cells and have gained recent attraction for this reason.[35] Furthermore, the growth properties of ASCs are superior to bone marrow–derived MSCs (BMSCs).[35] ASCs may be obtained either through liposuction aspirates or from the infrapatellar fat pad.[36] When cultured with appropriate growth factors (TGF-β, BMP-2, BMP-6, BMP-7), ASCs may differentiate into chondrocytes in vitro or in vivo.[37]

BMSCs are popular because of ease of collection (the procedure is minimally invasive) and the extensive laboratory characterization of these cells.[36,38] However, the cell yield is low following bone marrow aspiration, and therefore these stem cells often must be isolated and expanded in cell culture before clinical use. Common extraction sites are the iliac crest, the tibia, and the femur.[31] MSCs may differ between anatomic regions of the same tissue type in terms of yield and characteristics.[5] In the case of BMSCs, bone marrow is aspirated 3 weeks before the transplantation is set to occur. The aspirated cells are then cultured in a monolayer for expansion. Several factors can be used to induce these cells to differentiate into host mesenchymal tissue, including cartilage and bone. The cells can then be cultured in scaffolds to transplant into the affected joint. Synovial-derived MSCs have the most promising chondrogenic ability, but little literature exists exploring this topic.[31]

There are 2 methods of incorporation of MSCs into articular cartilage: (1) surgical implantation by embedding the cells in a scaffold, and (2) intra-articular injections.[38] Several animal models have been used to test the effects of matrix-assisted or scaffold-assisted MSC transplantation,[39,40] as well as intra-articular injection of MSCs[41] for the treatment of focal chondral defects, with overall successful results in terms of macroscopic and histologic observations. However, similar studies have not been conducted in human subjects with isolated cartilage defects.

In a case series of 18 patients with knee, ankle, or hip OA, Emadedin and colleagues[42] evaluated the effect of 1 intra-articular injection of approximately 5×10^5 cells/kg body weight of BMSCs. At a final follow-up of 30 months' posttransplantation, no serious adverse events were reported. Furthermore, no changes were observed in liver function, hematology, or biochemistry analyses. Walking distance, VAS for pain, and WOMAC scores all improved from baseline to final follow-up. In terms of imaging outcomes, reduced subchondral bone edema was appreciated in 3 of 6 patients with knee OA and 4 of 6 patients with ankle OA at 6-month follow-up. Articular cartilage repair was visualized with MRI in 3 of 5 patients with hip OA.

Results of a phase I clinical trial were recently published on the use of ASCs for the treatment of knee OA.[43] A consecutive series of 18 patients with severe knee OA were treated with a single intra-articular injection of autologous ASCs. To determine a potential dose-response relationship, patients were separated into 3 groups of 6 patients each: low dose (2×10^6 cells), medium dose (10×10^6 cells), and high dose (50×10^6 cells). At 6-month follow-up, no serious adverse events were reported, and even patients in the low-dose group experienced significant improvements in pain levels and function compared with baseline.

In another phase I-II clinical trial, Soler and colleagues[44] recently reported on 15 patients with knee OA (K-L grade II or III) who were treated with a single intra-articular injection of a mean 40.9×10^6 autologous BMSCs. At a follow-up of 12 months, 1 serious adverse event had been reported, a ruptured ovarian cyst, which was likely not related to the stem cell therapy. Compared with baseline, VAS pain score, the

Lequesne functional index, and the WOMAC score significantly improved at the 12-month follow-up (all $P = .001$). Furthermore, each of the following WOMAC subscales significantly improved between baseline and 12-month follow-up: pain ($P = .008$), stiffness ($P = .01$), and functionality ($P = .001$). Thirteen of the 15 patients were followed until 4 years' postinjection and assessed with the VAS, which revealed a further reduction in pain from the 12-month follow-up. Finally, MRI T2 mapping was performed to assess cartilage quality, with a steadily decreasing value observed from preinjection to 12-month follow-up, indicative of cartilage regeneration.

In a retrospective cohort study of patients undergoing arthroscopic procedures for knee OA, Kim and colleagues[45] compared outcomes of MSC injections in combination with PRP (n = 20) versus a matched pair of patients who underwent MSC implantation on a fibrin glue scaffold (n = 20). At a mean follow-up of 28.6 months, IKDC and Tegner activity scores significantly improved in both groups compared with preoperatively, with a significantly higher IKDC score in the implantation group. Although preliminary outcomes of cartilage treatment by BMSCs in the knee show no tumor growth or infection, long-term safety of stem cell therapy for articular cartilage therapy has yet to be proven.[38]

MSCs are an attractive option for patients with articular cartilage damage, as MSCs may differentiate into chondrocytes in the appropriate environment. Currently, published outcomes are mostly limited to phase I-II clinical trials, with their primary goal focused on the assessment of safety and tolerability of MSC transplantation. Further research is necessary to determine optimal harvest location, culture methods, cell concentration, and transplantation method. Although the intra-articular transplantation of MSCs has not been associated with severe adverse events, long-term follow-up is necessary before this therapy can be definitively considered safe and effective.

DISCUSSION

As awareness increases throughout the orthopedic community of the importance of treating early osteoarthritis and focal chondral defects, newer treatment modalities have been used in an attempt to prevent or delay progression to late-stage OA. Although successful surgical procedures exist, particularly for the treatment of isolated articular cartilage lesions, biological therapies carry the advantages of being less invasive and less expensive. Based on this review, few studies have reported outcomes of these treatment options in the management of knee and hip articular cartilage damage, although generally positive outcomes have been reported in these studies.

Although many of the studies discussed in this review have focused on the use of singular treatment methods, some of these options can and have been used in conjunction with each other. PRP has been used to augment BMAC therapy, although it is still unknown if these treatments result in a synergistic effect.[23]

There are a number of variables within each of the biological treatment options discussed in this review. As a result of the variability that exists within each of these treatment options, further research is necessary (1) to establish benchmarks for preparation and formulation of each biological therapy, and (2) to make comparisons between different biological options. For example, the viability and efficacy of BMAC or stem cell therapy likely is affected by harvest location, cell concentration, donor sex,[46,47] donor age,[47,48] and donor health.[49] Likewise, the effectiveness of PRP likely depends on leukocyte concentration.[9]

More research is necessary for all biological options described in this review to draw any definitive conclusions, especially in the realm of long-term effects. Most studies in the current literature include patients with knee OA, with few published studies demonstrating outcomes in patients with hip OA. BMAC appears as a promising option at present, as it is FDA-approved and has the benefits of including both stem cells and growth factors.[23] Although all biological options provide a viable alternative to surgery for patients, the long-term effects of these modalities are yet to be determined.

ACKNOWLEDGMENTS

The authors would like to acknowledge Abigail Richards for her assistance with the article preparation.

REFERENCES

1. Widuchowski W, Lukasik P, Kwiatkowski G, et al. Isolated full thickness chondral injuries. Prevalence and outcome of treatment. A retrospective study of 5233 knee arthroscopies. Acta Chir Orthop Traumatol Cech 2008;75(5):382–6.
2. Ciccotti MC, Kraeutler MJ, Austin LS, et al. The prevalence of articular cartilage changes in the knee joint in patients undergoing arthroscopy for meniscal pathology. Arthroscopy 2012;28(10):1437–44.
3. Murray IR, LaPrade RF. Platelet-rich plasma: Renewed scientific understanding must guide appropriate use. Bone Joint Res 2016;5(3):92–4.
4. Kraeutler MJ, Garabekyan T, Mei-Dan O. The use of platelet-rich plasma to augment conservative and surgical treatment of hip and pelvic disorders. Muscles Ligaments Tendons J 2016;6(3):410–9.
5. LaPrade RF, Dragoo JL, Koh JL, et al. AAOS research symposium updates and consensus: biologic treatment of orthopaedic injuries. J Am Acad Orthop Surg 2016;24(7):e62–78.
6. Fleming BC, Proffen BL, Vavken P, et al. Increased platelet concentration does not improve functional graft healing in bio-enhanced ACL reconstruction. Knee Surg Sports Traumatol Arthrosc 2015;23(4):1161–70.
7. Yoshida R, Cheng M, Murray MM. Increasing platelet concentration in platelet-rich plasma inhibits anterior cruciate ligament cell function in three-dimensional culture. J Orthop Res 2014;32(2):291–5.
8. Weibrich G, Hansen T, Kleis W, et al. Effect of platelet concentration in platelet-rich plasma on peri-implant bone regeneration. Bone 2004;34(4):665–71.
9. Riboh JC, Saltzman BM, Yanke AB, et al. Effect of leukocyte concentration on the efficacy of platelet-rich plasma in the treatment of knee osteoarthritis. Am J Sports Med 2016;44(3):792–800.
10. Patel S, Dhillon MS, Aggarwal S, et al. Treatment with platelet-rich plasma is more effective than placebo for knee osteoarthritis: a prospective, double-blind, randomized trial. Am J Sports Med 2013;41(2):356–64.
11. Cerza F, Carnì S, Carcangiu A, et al. Comparison between hyaluronic acid and platelet-rich plasma, intra-articular infiltration in the treatment of gonarthrosis. Am J Sports Med 2012;40(12):2822–7.
12. Sánchez M, Fiz N, Azofra J, et al. A randomized clinical trial evaluating plasma rich in growth factors (PRGF-Endoret) versus hyaluronic acid in the short-term treatment of symptomatic knee osteoarthritis. Arthroscopy 2012;28(8):1070–8.
13. Filardo G, Di Matteo B, Di Martino A, et al. Platelet-rich plasma intra-articular knee injections show no superiority versus viscosupplementation: a randomized controlled trial. Am J Sports Med 2015;43(7):1575–82.

14. Filardo G, Kon E, Di Martino A, et al. Platelet-rich plasma vs hyaluronic acid to treat knee degenerative pathology: study design and preliminary results of a randomized controlled trial. BMC Musculoskelet Disord 2012;13:229.

15. Wolfstadt JI, Cole BJ, Ogilvie-Harris DJ, et al. Current concepts: the role of mesenchymal stem cells in the management of knee osteoarthritis. Sports Health 2015;7(1):38–44.

16. Abrams GD, Frank RM, Fortier LA, et al. Platelet-rich plasma for articular cartilage repair. Sports Med Arthrosc 2013;21(4):213–9.

17. Duif C, Vogel T, Topcuoglu F, et al. Does intraoperative application of leukocyte-poor platelet-rich plasma during arthroscopy for knee degeneration affect postoperative pain, function and quality of life? A 12-month randomized controlled double-blind trial. Arch Orthop Trauma Surg 2015;135(7):971–7.

18. Dallari D, Stagni C, Rani N, et al. Ultrasound-guided injection of platelet-rich plasma and hyaluronic acid, separately and in combination, for hip osteoarthritis: a randomized controlled trial. Am J Sports Med 2016;44(3):664–71.

19. Battaglia M, Guaraldi F, Vannini F, et al. Efficacy of ultrasound-guided intra-articular injections of platelet-rich plasma versus hyaluronic acid for hip osteoarthritis. Orthopedics 2013;36(12):e1501–8.

20. Liu J, Song W, Yuan T, et al. A comparison between platelet-rich plasma (PRP) and hyaluronate acid on the healing of cartilage defects. PLoS One 2014;9(5): e97293.

21. Milano G, Deriu L, Sanna Passino E, et al. The effect of autologous conditioned plasma on the treatment of focal chondral defects of the knee. An experimental study. Int J Immunopathol Pharmacol 2011;24(1 Suppl 2):117–24.

22. Goodrich LR, Chen AC, Werpy NM, et al. Addition of mesenchymal stem cells to autologous platelet-enhanced fibrin scaffolds in chondral defects: does it enhance repair? J Bone Joint Surg Am 2016;98(1):23–34.

23. Chahla J, Dean CS, Moatshe G, et al. Concentrated bone marrow aspirate for the treatment of chondral injuries and osteoarthritis of the knee: a systematic review of outcomes. Orthop J Sports Med 2016;4(1):2325967115625481.

24. Kim JD, Lee GW, Jung GH, et al. Clinical outcome of autologous bone marrow aspirates concentrate (BMAC) injection in degenerative arthritis of the knee. Eur J Orthop Surg Traumatol 2014;24(8):1505–11.

25. Hauser RA, Orlofsky A. Regenerative injection therapy with whole bone marrow aspirate for degenerative joint disease: a case series. Clin Med Insights Arthritis Musculoskelet Disord 2013;6:65–72.

26. Hernigou P, Homma Y, Flouzat Lachaniette CH, et al. Benefits of small volume and small syringe for bone marrow aspirations of mesenchymal stem cells. Int Orthop 2013;37(11):2279–87.

27. Gobbi A, Karnatzikos G, Scotti C, et al. One-step cartilage repair with bone marrow aspirate concentrated cells and collagen matrix in full-thickness knee cartilage lesions: results at 2-year follow-up. Cartilage 2011;2(3):286–99.

28. Gobbi A, Scotti C, Karnatzikos G, et al. One-step surgery with multipotent stem cells and hyaluronan-based scaffold for the treatment of full-thickness chondral defects of the knee in patients older than 45 years. Knee Surg Sports Traumatol Arthrosc 2016. [Epub ahead of print].

29. Muschler GF, Midura RJ. Connective tissue progenitors: practical concepts for clinical applications. Clin Orthop Relat Res 2002;395:66–80.

30. Potten CS, Loeffler M. Stem cells: Attributes, cycles, spirals, pitfalls and uncertainties. Lessons for and from the crypt. Development 1990;110(4):1001–20.

31. Chang YH, Liu HW, Wu KC, et al. Mesenchymal stem cells and their clinical applications in osteoarthritis. Cell Transplant 2016;25(5):937–50.
32. Lietman SA. Induced pluripotent stem cells in cartilage repair. World J Orthop 2016;7(3):149–55.
33. Zlotnicki JP, Geeslin AG, Murray IR, et al. Biologic treatments for sports injuries II think tank-current concepts, future research, and barriers to advancement, Part 3: articular cartilage. Orthop J Sports Med 2016;4(4):2325967116642433.
34. Dominici M, Le Blanc K, Mueller I, et al. Minimal criteria for defining multipotent mesenchymal stromal cells. The International Society for Cellular Therapy position statement. Cytotherapy 2006;8(4):315–7.
35. Ruetze M, Richter W. Adipose-derived stromal cells for osteoarticular repair: trophic function versus stem cell activity. Expert Rev Mol Med 2014;16:e9.
36. LaPrade RF, Geeslin AG, Murray IR, et al. Biologic treatments for sports injuries II think tank–current concepts, future research, and barriers to advancement, Part 1: biologics overview, ligament injury, tendinopathy. Am J Sports Med 2016;44(12):3270–83.
37. Wu L, Cai X, Zhang S, et al. Regeneration of articular cartilage by adipose tissue derived mesenchymal stem cells: perspectives from stem cell biology and molecular medicine. J Cell Physiol 2013;228(5):938–44.
38. Filardo G, Madry H, Jelic M, et al. Mesenchymal stem cells for the treatment of cartilage lesions: from preclinical findings to clinical application in orthopaedics. Knee Surg Sports Traumatol Arthrosc 2013;21(8):1717–29.
39. Jang KM, Lee JH, Park CM, et al. Xenotransplantation of human mesenchymal stem cells for repair of osteochondral defects in rabbits using osteochondral biphasic composite constructs. Knee Surg Sports Traumatol Arthrosc 2014; 22(6):1434–44.
40. Jung M, Kaszap B, Redöhl A, et al. Enhanced early tissue regeneration after matrix-assisted autologous mesenchymal stem cell transplantation in full thickness chondral defects in a minipig model. Cell Transplant 2009;18(8):923–32.
41. Nam HY, Karunanithi P, Loo WC, et al. The effects of staged intra-articular injection of cultured autologous mesenchymal stromal cells on the repair of damaged cartilage: a pilot study in caprine model. Arthritis Res Ther 2013;15(5):R129.
42. Emadedin M, Ghorbani Liastani M, Fazeli R, et al. Long-term follow-up of intra-articular injection of autologous mesenchymal stem cells in patients with knee, ankle, or hip osteoarthritis. Arch Iran Med 2015;18(6):336–44.
43. Pers YM, Rackwitz L, Ferreira R, et al. Adipose mesenchymal stromal cell-based therapy for severe osteoarthritis of the knee: a Phase I dose-escalation trial. Stem Cells Transl Med 2016;5(7):847–56.
44. Soler R, Orozco L, Munar A, et al. Final results of a phase I-II trial using ex vivo expanded autologous mesenchymal stromal cells for the treatment of osteoarthritis of the knee confirming safety and suggesting cartilage regeneration. Knee 2016;23(4):647–54.
45. Kim YS, Kwon OR, Choi YJ, et al. Comparative matched-pair analysis of the injection versus implantation of mesenchymal stem cells for knee osteoarthritis. Am J Sports Med 2015;43(11):2738–46.
46. Matsumoto T, Kubo S, Meszaros LB, et al. The influence of sex on the chondrogenic potential of muscle-derived stem cells: implications for cartilage regeneration and repair. Arthritis Rheum 2008;58(12):3809–19.
47. Payne KA, Didiano DM, Chu CR. Donor sex and age influence the chondrogenic potential of human femoral bone marrow stem cells. Osteoarthritis Cartilage 2010;18(5):705–13.

48. Choudhery MS, Badowski M, Muise A, et al. Donor age negatively impacts adipose tissue-derived mesenchymal stem cell expansion and differentiation. J Transl Med 2014;12:8.
49. Chandran P, Le Y, Li Y, et al. Mesenchymal stromal cells from patients with acute myeloid leukemia have altered capacity to expand differentiated hematopoietic progenitors. Leuk Res 2015;39(4):486–93.

Management of Osteochondritis Dissecans Lesions of the Knee, Elbow and Ankle

Kathryn L. Bauer, MD[a], John D. Polousky, MD[b],*

KEYWORDS

- Osteochondritis dissecans • Articular cartilage • OCD • Arthroscopy • Microfracture
- Autologous chondrocyte implantation • Osteochondral allograft

KEY POINTS

- Osteochondritis dissecans (OCD) lesions involve destruction of the subchondral bone and overlying articular cartilage. The knee is the most common location, although the ankle and elbow are often involved.
- History and physical examination findings are often vague; therefore, diagnosis relies on proper interpretation of plain radiographs and MRI findings.
- There is currently no consensus regarding the optimal cartilage restoration techniques.
- Risk factors for OCD lesions requiring surgical management are age (skeletal maturity) and instability of the OCD fragment.

INTRODUCTION

Osteochondritis dissecans (OCD) has been defined as "a focal, idiopathic alteration of subchondral bone structure *with* risk for instability and disruption of adjacent articular cartilage that may result in premature osteoarthritis."[1] Although most often problematic in the knee, OCD lesions can affect the articular cartilage of the elbow and ankle as well.[2] The incidence of OCD lesions is unknown, primarily owing to inconsistencies in reported classification systems, criteria for diagnosis, and multiple options for available treatment.[3] There are multiple theories previously proposed regarding the etiology of OCD lesions in the knee, elbow, and ankle, including family history, local

Disclosure Statement: K.L. Bauer has nothing to disclose. Consultant: AlloSource, Joint Restoration Foundation; Board Member: ROCK Study Group (J.D. Polousky).
[a] Children's Health Andrews Institute for Orthopedics and Sports Medicine, 7601 Preston Road, Suite 3600, Plano, TX 75024, USA; [b] Children's Health Andrews Institute for Orthopedics and Sports Medicine, 7601 Preston Road, Suite P3608, Plano, TX 75024, USA
* Corresponding author.
E-mail address: John.Polousky@childrens.com

Clin Sports Med 36 (2017) 469–487
http://dx.doi.org/10.1016/j.csm.2017.02.005
0278-5919/17/© 2017 Elsevier Inc. All rights reserved.

ischemia, and trauma or repetitive microtrauma.[4–7] There are a variety of treatment options available, with decisions regarding treatment primarily hinging on patient skeletal age and stability of the OCD lesion. Owing to vague history and paucity of examination findings, diagnosis and management depend on proper interpretation of imaging studies. Treatment options range from immobilization, rest from activity, and bracing to surgical interventions, including loose body removal, arthroscopic fixation of an unstable fragment, or more invasive drilling and cartilage restoration procedures. Diagnostic and treatment options based on the current available literature for OCD lesions of the knee, elbow and ankle are outlined herein.

KNEE
Patient Evaluation: History and Physical Examination

Patients with OCD lesions of the knee often have 1 of 2 different presentations. Frequently, the OCD is found as an incidental finding while the child is being evaluated for knee pain as the result of a different injury.[8] Other patients present with vague knee pain after activity, with or without a mild limp, and often do not report a specific history of trauma.[9] It is not until the stability of the fragment is compromised, or even completely detached, that mechanical symptoms of locking, popping, and catching are reported. A knee effusion is rarely encountered, and will be seen in less than 20% of patients upon presentation.[10] Owing to the typically mild initial symptoms, patients often have prolonged pain before first seeking help for their condition. Cahill and Ahten[9] reported that the majority of their patients had pain for up to 14 months upon initial presentation.

In 1967, Wilson[11] described a physical examination finding to aid in diagnosis of OCD lesion. With this maneuver, the knee is placed in 90° of flexion. As the tibia is rotated externally, the knee will be extended to 30° of flexion. Pain at the anteromedial aspect of the knee is considered a positive test, and the knee pain will subside with internal rotation of the tibia. The pain experienced is thought to be the result of impingement of the tibial spine on the lateral aspect of the medial femoral condyle, the most common location for OCD in the knee. This test is not helpful in cases where lesions are not in the "classic" location, and in fact the test has little diagnostic usefulness,[12] because it has been found to be positive in only 16% of knees with diagnosed OCD lesions.[10]

Imaging

Because the history and physical examination findings are nonspecific, the diagnosis of an OCD lesion is reliant on imaging modalities. If proper views are obtained, the presence of most OCD lesions can be diagnosed with plain radiographs (**Fig. 1**). Four specific views of the knee are recommended including the standard anteroposterior (AP) and lateral images, as well as a 45° flexed tunnel view and merchant view.[13] This combination provides visualization of the most common locations of OCD lesions in the knee. Additionally, because many patients will have bilateral involvement,[2,9] it is sometimes advocated to obtain radiographs of the contralateral side as well. An OCD lesion on plain imaging will show a well-defined area of subchondral bone separated by a sclerotic rim outlining the fragment.[14] Plain radiographs also help to determine the skeletal maturity of the patient, which is important, because patients with open physes have a better prognosis.[2]

Although useful to establish the presence of an OCD lesion, it is difficult to establish stability of the lesion based on plain radiographs alone.[14] MRI is currently considered the imaging modality of choice to evaluate the location, size and, stability of the OCD

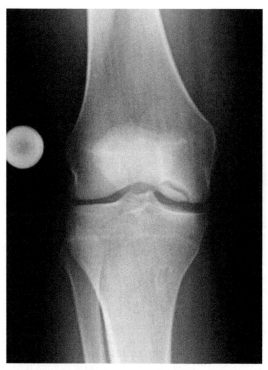

Fig. 1. Plain radiograph demonstrating an osteochondritis dissecans lesion in the medial femoral condyle.

lesion[14] (**Fig. 2**). Stability of an OCD lesion is defined as the presence or absence of separation of the osteochondral fragment from the underlying parent bone.[15] DeSmet and coworkers established 4 criteria found on T2-weighted MRI studies to help define instability of the fragment verified by arthroscopy. These findings included (1) high-intensity signal beneath the OCD lesion, (2) a well-defined focal defect in the overlying articular cartilage, (3) fracture of the overlying articular cartilage, and (4) subchondral cysts.[16,17] The most predictive factor of instability was the presence of a high-intensity signal line between the lesion and the underlying "normal" bone. Accuracy of predicting instability on MRI can be increased to 85% when the criteria includes not only high signal line present on T2 images, but also the presence of fracture of the articular cartilage on T1 images.[18] Kijowski and colleagues[19] evaluated the sensitivity and specificity of the criteria DeSmet proposed with regard to predicting arthroscopic instability, where instability is defined as visualized evidence of articular cartilage disruption or obvious motion of the articular cartilage of the OCD lesion. In this study, when all 4 criteria defined previously by DeSmet were present, there was 100% sensitivity and specificity for instability in adult OCD lesions. In juvenile OCD (JOCD), however, the sensitivity remained 100%, but the specificity decreased to 11%.[19] The use of MRI studies to evaluate the stability of the lesion has again been shown to be more predictable in patients with closed physes than in those with JOCD lesions, where a high number of lesions were classified as unstable based on MRI findings but were in fact stable on arthroscopy in a recent article by Heywood and associates.[20] MRI scanning is useful to identify the presence of loose fragments as well (**Fig. 3**).

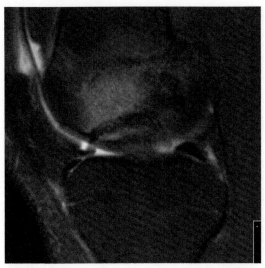

Fig. 2. MRI scan demonstrating an unstable osteochondritis dissecans lesion. Note the disruption in the articular surface and subchondral bone.

Nonsurgical Treatment

Recently proposed treatment algorithms are based primarily on the stability of an OCD lesion and skeletal maturity.[3,10] Multiple classification schemes have been established for OCD lesions, with all including stability and skeletal maturity as key factors in decision making.[4,16,17] Nonoperative management is often recommended as a first-line treatment for stable OCD lesions in skeletally immature patients (JOCD).[14,21] Improved prognosis has been reported in young patients with lesion where the articular cartilage remains intact, lesions size is less than 2 cm^2, and lesions in the classic

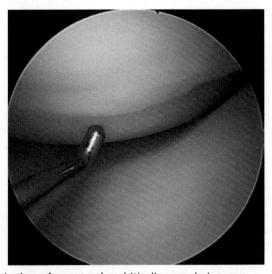

Fig. 3. Arthroscopic view of an osteochondritis dissecans lesion.

location on the lateral aspect of the MFC.[10] Wall and colleagues[21] noted that 66% of patients with JOCD lesions progressed to healing with up to 6 months of nonoperative treatment, including activity modification and immobilization.[21] It was noted in their study as well that larger lesions and mechanical symptoms consistent with instability were less likely to heal.

Surgical Treatment

Unstable OCD lesions and stable lesions that fail to respond to nonoperative management progress to surgical intervention. Lesions found on the lateral femoral condyle (40.3%) are more likely to progress to surgery than those found in the classic location on the medial femoral condyle (28.2%); as was reported previously, the classical location tends to have a better prognosis.[2,10] It has also been estimated that 58.5% of all OCD lesions requiring surgical management occur in the knee, and those patients who are nearing skeletal maturity are 7.4 times more likely to progress to surgery than those under age 11 years.[2] Surgical treatment varies depending on surgeon preference and patient factors.

Retroarticular/transarticular drilling

Arthroscopic drilling is indicated in stable lesions that fail nonoperative treatment. Drilling may be either retroarticular (also known as extraarticular or intraepiphyseal; this does not violate the articular cartilage; **Fig. 4**) or transarticular (also termed transchondral). Rates of healing vary according to various studies, and interpreting the data is further complicated by varying definitions of healing depending on author. In 2001, Kocher and colleagues[8] described significant improvements in function and 100% rate of radiographic healing in patients treated with transarticular arthroscopic drilling. Donaldson and Wojtys[22] reported 92.3% of skeletally immature knees treated with retroarticular drilling of stable lesions to have excellent outcomes at an average of 8.5 months postoperatively. In this study results, were based on return to activity, normal physical examination, and improvement of appearance of lesion on

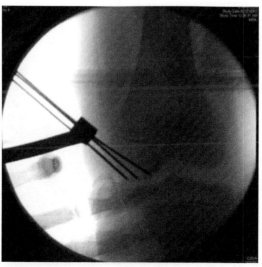

Fig. 4. Intraoperative fluoroscopy image of retroarticular drilling of a stable osteochondritis dissecans lesion.

radiographs.[22] Adachi and colleagues[23] reported a 95% healing rate in JOCD treated with retroarticular drilling as evaluated with both plain radiographs and MRI. Additionally, they showed significant functional improvement by use of Lysholm scores. Edmonds and colleagues[24] also showed a mean rate of radiographic healing to be 98.2% for retroarticular drilling at final follow-up. They also found that large OCD lesions took almost twice as long to heal when compared with smaller lesions.

A recent systematic review of the literature by Gunton and colleagues[25] compared retroarticular and transarticular drilling, finding comparable results between the 2 modalities. Radiographic healing occurred in 86% of those drilled retroarticularly compared with 91% treated with transarticular drilling. There were no reported surgical complications with either modality, although retroarticular drilling is thought to be more challenging technically and requires the use of fluoroscopy.[15,24,25]

In situ fixation

When the articular cartilage is unstable, surgical fixation is indicated. Many different fixation techniques have been described, including metallic headed screws, metallic headless compression screws, bioabsorbable implants, and osteochondral plugs. Lesions with substantial bone stock remaining are suitable for screw fixation, with several authors showing high rates of healing 88% to 100%.[26–29] Kocher and colleagues[30] showed an 84.6% rate of healing in 26 JOCD lesions treated with varying fixation methods, including variable pitch screws, bioabsorbable tacks, partially threaded cannulated screws, and bioabsorbable pins. They also showed 100% healing rate in fixation of completely detached lesions. Magnussen and colleagues[31] reported 92% stable healing in patients with unstable grade IV OCD lesions treated with metallic fixation. Metallic screws, especially headed screws, are removed, requiring a second procedure at 6 to 12 weeks after implantation. This offers a chance for a "second look" to assess healing of the lesion[15] (**Fig. 5**).

Bioabsorbable implants, including pins, darts, or screws, have been used with success as well.[30,32–34] These implants have the potential benefit of not requiring a second surgery for removal and provide no interference during postoperative MRI

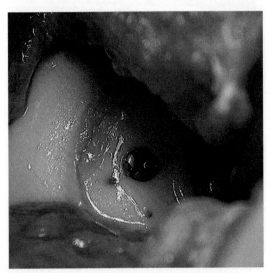

Fig. 5. Fixation of an osteochondritis dissecans lesion with metallic screws.

evaluation.[26,34] Use of a Poly 96L/4D-lactide copolymer bioabsorbable implant showed MRI evidence of healing in 94.1% of patients, and good to excellent clinical outcome in 22 of 24 skeletally immature patients.[34] Skeletally mature patients treated with fixation with bioabsorbable fixation seem to have a lower rate of healing and higher complication rate. Complications included loose body formation in 33% and 18% reoperation rate for implant backout.[35] Other investigators have also shown complications with bioabsorbable fixation methods, including damage of the opposing articular cartilage, implant breakage with loose body formation, and cyst formation.[36]

Biologic fixation of OCD lesions is being explored as well, with the use of osteochondral plugs for fixation of the lesion.[37–40] In 2007, Miniaci and Tytherleigh-Strong[40] described a series of patients treated with multiple 4.5-mm osteochondral autograft plugs that reported visual analog pain scores of 0 out of 10 at the 1-year follow-up. This was a significant reduction compared with their preoperative average score of 8.3 out of 10. Additionally, they showed complete bony incorporation in all knees at 6 months postoperatively, and healing of the cartilage component at 9 months.[40]

Debridement with or without microfracture

In cases of fragmentation of the OCD lesion or poor quality of the cartilage (either significant loss leading to incongruity or deep fissuring), the fragment is not repairable and should be excised. Further treatment after excision is based on the individual characteristics of the patient and lesion, as well as surgeon preference. Excision of the fragment in isolation is not recommended typically. Although there may be short-term improvement in pain and function, long-term results are poor, with a 29% rate of radiographic healing and a high rate (79%) of degenerative changes on plain radiographs at a mean of 11 years of follow-up.[41,42]

The role of microfracture in OCD lesions is less defined when compared with its use in traumatic chondral defects.[15] One prospective, randomized study that compared microfracture with osteochondral allograft treatment showed significant initial improvement in symptoms; however, 41% of the microfracture group showed decline at 4 years leading to a second surgery based on pain and effusions, compared with 0% in the transplant group.[43]

Autologous chondrocyte implantation has also been used in conjunction with fragment debridement.[44,45] Peterson and colleagues[44] reported a 93% improvement in patient self-assessment questionnaires in a mixture of JOCD and adult OCD treated with autologous chondrocyte implantation with a mean follow-up of 5.6 years. Two patients in their study reported failure of treatment in the early postoperative period.

Osteochondral autograft or allograft transplantation

Osteochondral autograft and allograft transplantation has been used in both traumatic chondral injuries and the treatment of irreparable OCD lesions.[43,46–49] Lyon and colleagues[48] have shown osteochondral allografts to be a viable treatment option JOCD. In this study, they found full return to sporting activities at 9 to 12 months postoperatively and complete radiographic incorporation of the allograft at the 2-year follow-up. Other authors have also shown success with fresh osteochondral allograft in both juvenile and adult patients with type III or IV OCD lesions, with clinical outcomes in 72% rated as "good to excellent"[49] (**Fig. 6**).

ELBOW
Patient Evaluation

The capitellum is the most common site of OCD lesion in the elbow. This pathology is typically seen in young athletes involved in overhand throwing or weight-bearing

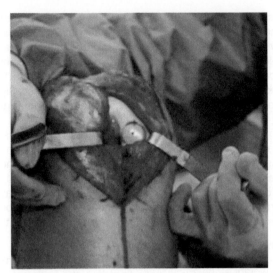

Fig. 6. Osteochondral allograft transplantation for an unsalvageable osteochondritis dissecans lesion.

activities; adults are rarely affected.[50,51] Because they are thought to arise from repetitive trauma causing local ischemia to the subchondral bone during overhead activities, the dominant arm is affected more often.[52,53] OCD lesions can occur in the radial head, trochlea, or olecranon, but are significantly less common in these locations.[54,55] The portion of the capitellum involved is usually the area that engages the radial head at around 45° of elbow flexion.[56]

Patients typically present with activity-related pain in the elbow that gradually worsens over time.[57] Specific trauma is not reported typically. Similar to the knee, patients may complain of mechanical symptoms, including catching, popping, or locking. The presence of mechanical symptoms raises suspicion for loose bodies in the joint.[58] Patients report lateral elbow pain and have tenderness located at the radiocapitellar joint. Loss of range of motion can be present, with loss seen in both flexion and extension; loss of extension is slightly more common.[59] Patients may demonstrate a positive radiocapitellar compression test with pain during active supination and pronation while the elbow is extended.[60]

First-line imaging includes 3 views with plane radiographs of the elbow, including an AP with the elbow extended, lateral elbow radiograph, and a 45° flexion AP.[58] In cases of early OCD lesions, plain radiographs may be negative; in fact, only 66% of patients with a known OCD of the capitellum have positive findings on initial plain radiographs.[61] Changes at the anterolateral aspect of the capitellum include subchondral lucency or sclerosis, flattening of the capitellum, or fragmentation.[58,60] Patients with OCD of the capitellum should be distinguished from those with Panner's disease. Panner's disease is an atraumatic, idiopathic osteochondrosis of the capitellum affecting children 10 years of age or younger.[58,60] This condition is self-limiting, and is treated conservatively with rest from painful activities, antiinflammatory drugs, with or without a brief period of immobilization. Patients typically return to previous activity level around 8 weeks once symptoms have resolved. Follow-up radiographs show reossification as symptoms resolve.[58] In contrast with patients with Panner's disease, those with OCD of the capitellum are typically older adolescents.[51,58,60]

MRI scanning is currently the modality of choice to evaluate OCD of the capitellum, because plain radiographs have poor interobserver reliability.[62,63] Because early stage OCD lesions may present without findings on plane radiographs, MRI scanning can be used to detect these lesions.[58,60,64] Early stage lesions may present with normal signal on T2-weighted imaging, with only low signal intensity at the superficial capitellum seen on T1-weighted sequences. In more advanced stage OCD, changes will be seen on both T1-weighted and T2-weighted sequences (**Figs. 7** and **8**).[58,60,64] Kijowski and DeSmet[61] found that unstable lesions had both a thin line of high signal intensity between the lesion and the underlying parent bone and a round high-signal cyst on T2 sequences. These criteria were later revisited by Jans and colleagues,[65] who found that MRI was 100% sensitive for detecting an unstable lesion when 4 criteria were present: subchondral cyst, a fluid-filled defect underlying the OCD, high signal rim on T2-weighted imaging, and a high signal fracture line on T2-weighted images.

OCD of the capitellum has been classified based on both the status of the articular cartilage, as well as the stability of the subchondral bone. A common grading system cited by Lewine and colleagues[59] is listed below, although other classification systems exist.

- Grade I: articular surface and subchondral bone remain stable, localized softening present.
- Grade II: articular surface breech, stable subchondral bone.
- Grade III: articular surface breech, subchondral bone instability ("unstable in situ").
- Grade IV: detachment of OCD with loose body formation (**Fig. 9**).

Nonsurgical Treatment

The primary factor for determining treatment plan is stability of the capitellar OCD. Patients with stable lesions typically have an open capitellar physis, no fragmentation on imaging, and minimal loss of range of motion on examination.[66] Nonoperative

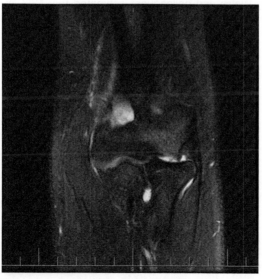

Fig. 7. Coronal MRI scan of an osteochondritis dissecans lesion in the capitellum of the elbow. Note the chondral defect and significant bone edema.

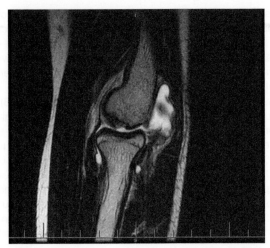

Fig. 8. Sagittal MRI image of a capitellar osteochondritis dissecans lesion. Note the disruption of the articular surface. The sagittal image often provides the best view of the lesion.

management includes immediate strict rest from aggravating activities involving the elbow.[58,67] Physical therapy is initiated to preserve range of motion, with strengthening being reserved until after complete resolution of symptoms. Throwing or weight bearing may gradually resume at 3 to 4 months if pain has resolved and range of motion is returned. Release to full activities is typically at 6 months if the patient remains asymptomatic. Patients with stable OCD lesions who are compliant with this protocol have been found to have an 84.2% healing rate. This decreases to 22.7% in patients who fail to comply.[68]

Surgical Treatment

A recent study by Weiss and colleagues[2] estimated that 12% of OCD lesions are found in the elbow, with 55% going on to require surgical treatment. Takahara and

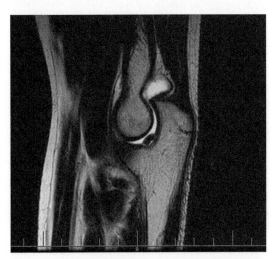

Fig. 9. Sagittal MRI demonstrating a loose body trapped in the ulno–humeral articulation.

colleagues[66] determined that unstable OCD lesions had a better long-term prognosis with surgical treatment when compared with nonoperative management. He classified these as patients with a closed capitellar physis, fragmentation of the OCD seen on plain imaging, and lack of range of motion measuring 20° or more. Surgical treatment is recommended in patients who continue to have symptoms with conservative management, loose bodies leading to mechanical symptoms, or unstable lesions as described elsewhere in this article.[59,60] Many surgical treatment options have been described; the decision as to which procedure to use depends on size of the OCD, stability of the overlying articular cartilage, and amount of extension to the lateral capitellum.[58,66] Lesions are considered "uncontained" if they extend past the lateral column of the distal humerus.[69] A recent study by Shi and colleagues[69] showed that at mean follow-up of 19.5 months patients with uncontained lesions had a greater flexion contracture. Mihara and colleagues[70] also described the importance of restoring the lateral aspect of the capitellum to achieve good clinical results.

Arthroscopic loose body removal with abrasion chondroplasty

Arthroscopy with loose body removal and abrasion chondroplasty to create a stable cartilage rim has been found to have better results in patients with smaller lesions (<50% of the capitellar surface involved) and those that do not involve the lateral column of the capitellum, or "contained" lesions.[58,66,69,71] Arthrotomy is sometimes necessary to remove large loose bodies after arthroscopy.[72]

Microfracture, antegrade drilling, and retrograde drilling

Many studies have reported good outcomes with regard to pain relief with arthroscopic debridement and microfracture.[50,51,59,72,73] Patients with OCD lesions of the capitellum treated with arthroscopic drilling can experience significant improvement in range of motion (both flexion and extension), with up to 86% returning to preinjury level of sports participation in 1 series.[72] A recent study by Lewine and colleagues[59] of adolescent patients with grade IV lesions treated with arthroscopic debridement and microfracture or drilling showed either clinical or radiographic resolution of the lesion in 71%, with 85.7% returning to any sport and 66.7% returning to their original sport. Nine patients complained of persistent mechanical symptoms and 4 patients in this study developed recurrent loose body formation after surgery.

In situ fracture fixation

In situ fixation of an unstable OCD lesion can be performed either arthroscopically or through an arthrotomy. Multiple modes of fixation have been reported, including metallic or absorbable headless compression screws, bioabsorbable pins, bone pegs, and Kirshner wires.[58] If significant subchondral bone stock has been lost, bone graft is placed under the lesion for support. In 2015, Hennrikus and associates[74] reported healing of elbow OCD lesions in 76.9% of patients who underwent internal fixation. Patients older than 15 years of age or those with thickness greater than 13 mm did not heal. Range of motion improved postoperatively by a mean of 18°.[74]

Recently, Uchida and coworkers[75] published the results of a cohort of 18 adolescent baseball players treated with arthroscopic fragment fixation with hydroxyapatite–poly-L-lactic acid thread pins. All but 1 patient healed, and 15 of 18 returned to the same or higher level of sport. Significant improvements were seen in both elbow flexion and extension. The 1 patient that who not achieve union underwent revision arthroscopy more than 1 year after surgery when fragmentation occurred.[75]

Osteochondral autograft

In cases where fragment fixation is not possible for unstable lesions, either owing to quality of the cartilage or lesion size, osteochondral transplantation is the next line of treatment.[58] Lesions involving greater than 50% of the articular surface of the capitellum are typically indicated for an osteochondral autograft transplantation system.[60,66] The donor site is typically a non–weight-bearing portion of the knee accessed via a small arthrotomy, and the recipient site is accessed via an anconeus split approach[56] or arthroscopically[76] and prepared with a coring reamer to a depth of 10 mm. The donor plug is then gently impacted in the recipient site until it is flush with surrounding articular cartilage.[56] When donor sites are kept at 10 mm in diameter or less, there is little or no resultant knee pain.[71,77–79]

Lyons and colleagues[78] recently published data on a cohort of 11 adolescent patients with capitellar OCD lesions greater than 1 cm^2 treated with an osteochondral autograft transplantation system that showed excellent results. All patients returned to their preoperative level of sport participation at an average of 4.4 months. Additionally, range of motion increased significantly with regard to both flexion and extension. Maruyama and colleagues[77] showed similar results, with 91% of patients pain free after surgery, and significantly improved range of motion. All patients showed graft incorporation on radiographs by 3.8 months. In this series, 93.9% of patients returned to their preoperative level of activity at a mean of 6.9 months. In this study, 1 patient did report mild activity-related anterior knee pain at the donor site.

Costal osteochondral autograft transplant

Recently, costal osteochondral transplantation has been advocated as a viable treatment option for lateral column OCD lesions of the elbow.[80,81] Nishinaka and colleagues[81] published results of 22 young patients treated with costal osteochondral transplantation. All patients in this study returned to their full preoperative activity level at a mean of 7.5 months. Four patients in this study did require unplanned return to the operating room for screw removal, loose body removal, and removal of spur formation.[81] Shimada and colleagues[80] similarly found good functional outcomes, with all patients treated with this technique achieving osseous union within 3 months. Similar to the previous study, 5 patients required additional surgery, including screw removal, loose body removal, and removal of spur formation.

ANKLE
Patient Evaluation

Kappis first described these lesions in the ankle joint in 1922.[82] Similar to the knee and elbow, OCD lesions of the ankle typically presents with vague, activity-related ankle pain. As with other locations described, mechanical symptoms of catching and locking may be present with unstable lesions. Patients typically do not present with a known history of trauma or injury, although displacement of a preexisting OCD fragment can occur after a traumatic injury. In fact, it is estimated that only 6.5% of OCD lesions of the talus become symptomatic after an ankle sprain.[83] It is important to differentiate OCD lesions from osteochondral fractures of the talus, which can be seen in traumatic settings and are considered to be a separate entity. Traumatic fractures are more often seen on the lateral aspect of the talus,[84] in contrast with the classic location for ankle OCD on the medial talar dome. True OCD lesions can be seen in the lateral or posterior talus, as well as the distal tibial plafond.

As compared with the knee and elbow that typically present in a younger population, OCD of the talus are often diagnosed with greater frequency in older adolescents and young adults, likely owing to a longer asymptomatic period.[85] Female patients seem to have a greater incidence of OCD of the ankle. There is a 6.9 times increased risk for ankle OCD in patients aged 12 to 19 years when compared with children aged 6 to 11 years of age.[86]

On examination, patients may report localized tenderness at the tibiotalar joint. Crepitus may be felt with passive range of motion of the ankle. Ligamentous stability should be examined. After the physical examination, radiographs of the ankle are obtained, including standard AP, mortise and lateral views. A subchondral "halo" can often be seen on the AP or mortise view. MRI studies as with other locations are used to evaluate stability and size, and to characterize location of the lesion. Detached OCD lesions on T2-weighted sequences will show a hyperintense line at the base of the lesion (**Figs. 10** and **11**).[87]

Nonsurgical Treatment

Treatment of OCD lesions of the ankle depends on patient age, and the stability and severity of symptoms. Stable lesions are typically treated conservatively. Short leg cast placement is recommended for 6 to 8 weeks, followed by activity restrictions for up to 6 months.[84] Young patients seem to have a greater healing potential with conservative treatment; therefore, in patients 12 years of age or younger, some have suggested continuing conservative treatment of for up to 1 year.[88] Perumal and colleagues[89] found that, after 6 months of conservative treatment, only 16% of their patients with a mean age of 11.9 years obtained clinical and radiographic healing. After 6 additional months of conservative treatment (1 year in total), an additional 46% obtained clinical healing. Nonoperative management in adults seems to be successful in fewer than one-half of cases.[84]

Surgical Treatment

Indications for surgical treatment include failure of conservative treatment with stable OCD, unstable OCD, and fragment detachment/loose body formation. Location of talar dome OCD lesions does not seem to strongly affect progression to surgical

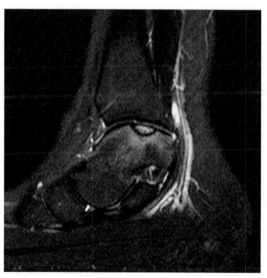

Fig. 10. Sagittal MRI image of an osteochondritis dissecans lesion in the talus. Note the extensive bony edema.

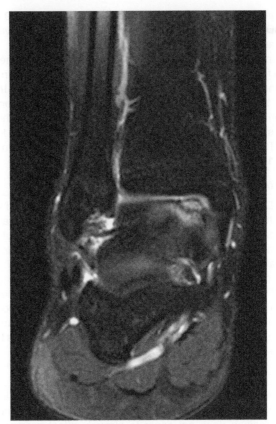

Fig. 11. Coronal MRI image of an osteochondritis dissecans (OCD) lesion in the talus. The medial shoulder of the talus is a common location for OCD.

treatment, although it may affect the treatment modality chosen.[2] Multiple treatment options are available with indications similar to those described in the knee and elbow:

- Arthroscopic or open debridement, loose body removal, with or without marrow stimulation.
- Fixation, with or without bone grafting.
- Transarticular drilling/retroarticular drilling.
- Autologous chondrocyte implantation.
- Osteochondral autograft/allograft transplantation.

Kramer and colleagues[90] recently reviewed 109 ankle OCD lesions and in this study found that the medial talus was the most common site requiring surgical treatment (73%). Procedures varied and included transarticular drilling, fragment fixation, or excision of an unstable fragment with microfracture. Reoperation rate was considered high at 27%. They determined female sex and elevated body mass index were negative predictors for outcome scores.

SUMMARY

Despite having been a recognized condition for more than 100 years, OCD remains a poorly understood disease of uncertain etiology. In general terms, OCD lesions, regardless of location, can be classified as stable or unstable. Similarly, OCD patients can be classified into 2 dichotomous groups: skeletally mature and skeletally immature. Nonoperative treatments of activity restriction and immobilization should be reserved for skeletally immature patients who have stable lesions, based on MRI studies. Operative intervention should be considered if the lesion does not demonstrate progress toward healing after 6 month of treatment.

Nonoperative treatment has demonstrated limited success in the treatment of unstable lesions in all age groups and in stable lesions in patients at or near skeletal maturity. In these groups, operative treatment should be considered as a first-line therapy. Operative options range from simple drilling and debridement techniques to advanced cartilage restoration, such as autologous chondrocyte implantation and osteochondral allografting.

REFERENCES

1. Edmonds EW, Shea KG. Osteochondritis dissecans: editorial comment. Clin Orthop Relat Res 2013;471(4):1105–6.
2. Weiss JM, Nikizad H, Shea KG, et al. The incidence of surgery in osteochondritis dissecans in children and adolescents. Orthop J Sports Med 2016;4(3):1–7.
3. Chambers HG, Shea KG, Carey JL. AAOS Clinical Practice Guideline: diagnosis and treatment of osteochondritis dissecans. J Am Acad Orthop Surg 2011;19(5): 307–9.
4. Cahill BR. Osteochondritis dissecans of the knee: treatment of juvenile and adult forms. J Am Acad Orthop Surg 1995;3(4):237–47.
5. Mubarak SJ, Carrol NC. Juvenile osteochondritis dissecans of the knee: etiology. Clin Orthop Relat Res 1981;157:200–11.
6. Bramer JA, Maas M, Dallinga RJ, et al. Increased external tibial torsion and osteochondritis dissecans of the knee. Clin Orthop Relat Res 2004;422:175–9.
7. Konig F. The classic: on loose bodies in the joint. Clin Orthop Relat Res 2013; 471(4):1107–15.
8. Kocher MS, Micheli LJ, Yaniv M, et al. Functional and radiographic outcomes of juvenile osteochondritis dissecans of the knee treated with transarticular arthroscopic drilling. Am J Sports Med 2001;29(5):562–6.
9. Cahill BR, Ahten SM. The three critical components in the conservative treatment of juvenile osteochondritis dissecans (JOCD). Physician, parent and child. Clin Sports Med 2001;20(2):287–98.
10. Hefti F, Beguiristain J, Krauspe R, et al. Osteochondritis dissecans: a multicenter study of the European Pediatric Orthopedic Society. J Pediatr Orthop B 1999; 8(4):231–45.
11. Wilson J. A diagnostic sign in osteochondritis dissecans of the knee. J Bone Joint Surg Am 1967;49(3):477–80.
12. Conrad J, Stanitski C. Osteochondritis dissecans: Wilson's sign revisited. Am J Sports Med 2003;31(5):777–8.
13. Crawford DC, Safran MR. Osteochondritis Dissecans of the Knee. J Am Acad Orthop Surg 2006;14(2):90–100.
14. Pascual-Garrido C, Moran CJ, Green DW, et al. Osteochondritis dissecans of the knee in children and adolescents. Curr Opin Pediatr 2013;25(1):46–51.
15. Edmonds EW, Polousky J. A review of knowledge in osteochondritis dissecans: 123 years of minimal evolution from Konig to the ROCK study group. Clin Orthop Relat Res 2013;471(4):1118–26.

16. DeSmet AA, Fisher DR, Graf BK, et al. Osteochondritis dissecans of the knee: value of MR imaging in determining lesion stability and the presence of articular cartilage defects. AJR Am J Roentgenol 1990;155:549–53.

17. DeSmet AA, Ilahi OA, Graf BK. Reassessment of the MR criteria for stability of osteochondritis dissecans in the knee and ankle. Skeletal Radiol 1996;25(2): 159–63.

18. O'Connor M, Palaniappan M, Khan N, et al. Osteochondritis dissecans of the knee in children. A comparison of MRI and arthroscopic findings. Bone Joint J 2002;84-B:2.

19. Kijowski R, Blankenbaker DG, Shinki K, et al. Juvenile versus adult osteochondritis dissecans of the knee: appropriate MR imaging criteria for instability. Radiology 2008;248(2):571–8.

20. Heywood CS, Benke MT, Brindle K, et al. Correlation of magnetic resonance imaging to arthroscopic findings of stability in juvenile osteochondritis dissecans. Arthroscopy 2011;27(2):194–9.

21. Wall EJ, Vourazeris J, Myer GD, et al. The healing potential of stable juvenile osteochondritis dissecans knee lesions. J Bone Joint Surg Am 2008;90(12): 2655–64.

22. Donaldson L, Wojtys E. Extraarticular drilling for stable osteochondritis dissecans in the skeletally immature knee. J Pediatr Orthop 2008;28(8):831–5.

23. Adachi N, Masataka D, Nakamae A, et al. Functional and radiographic outcome of stable juvenile osteochondritis dissecans of the knee treated with retroarticular drilling without bone grafting. Arthroscopy 2009;25(2):145–52.

24. Edmonds E, Albright J, Bastrom T, et al. Outcomes of extra-articular, intra-epiphyseal drilling for osteochondritis dissecans of the knee. J Pediatr Orthop 2010; 30(8):870–8.

25. Gunton M, Carey J, Shaw C, et al. Drilling Juvenile osteochondritis dissecans: retro- or transarticular. Clin Orthop Relat Res 2013;471(4):1144–51.

26. Makino A, Muscolo DL, Puigdevall M, et al. Arthroscopic fixation of osteochondritis dissecans of the knee: clinical, magnetic resonance imaging, and arthroscopic follow-up. Am J Sports Med 2005;33(10):1499–504.

27. Kouzelis A, Plessas S, Papadopoulos AX, et al. Herbert screw fixation and reverse guided drillings, for treatment of types III and IV osteochondritis dissecans. Knee Surg Sports Traumatol Arthrosc 2006;14(1):70–5.

28. Mackie I, Pemberton D, Maheson M. Arthroscopic use of the Herbert screw in osteochondritis dissecans. J Bone Joint Surg Br 1990;72(6):1076.

29. Thompson N. Osteochondritis dissecans and osteochondral fragments managed by Herbert compression screw fixation. Clin Orthop Relat Res 1987;224:71–8.

30. Kocher M, Czarnecki J, Andersen J, et al. Internal fixation of juvenile osteochondritis dissecans lesions of the knee. Am J Sports Med 2007;35(5):712–8.

31. Magnussen R, Carey J, Spindler K. Does operative fixation of an osteochondritis dissecans loose body result in healing and long-term maintenance of knee function. Am J Sports Med 2009;37(4):754–9.

32. Larsen M, Pietrzak W, DeLee J. Fixation of osteochondritis dissecans lesions using poly(l-lactic acid)/poly(glycolic acid) copolymer bioabsorbable screws. Am J Sports Med 2005;33(1):68–76.

33. Dines J, Fealy S, Potter H, et al. Outcomes of osteochondral lesions of the knee repaired with a bioabsorbable device. Arthroscopy 2008;24(1):62–8.

34. Tabaddor R, Banffy M, Michael B, et al. Fixation of juvenile osteochondritis dissecans lesions of the knee using poly 96L/4D-lactide copolymer bioabsorbable implants. J Pediatr Orthop 2010;30(1):14–20.

35. Millington K, Shah J, Dahm D, et al. Bioabsorbable fixation of unstable osteo-chondritis dissecans lesions. Am J Sports Med 2010;38(10):2065–70.
36. Friederichs M, Greis P, Burks R. Pitfalls associated with fixation of osteochondritis dissecans fragments using bioabsorbable screws. Arthroscopy 2001;17(5): 542–5.
37. Kobayashi T, Fujikawa K, Oohashi M. Surgical fixation of massive osteochondritis dissecans lesion using cylindrical osteochondral plugs. Arthroscopy 2004;20(9): 981–6.
38. Fonesca F, Balaco I. Fixation with autogenous osteochondral grafts for the treat-ment of osteochondritis dissecans (stages III and IV). Int Orthop 2009;33(1): 139–44.
39. Miura K, Ishibashi Y, Tsuda E, et al. Results of arthroscopic fixation of osteochon-dritis dissecans lesion of the knee with cylindrical autogenous osteochondral plugs. Am J Sports Med 2007;35(2):216–22.
40. Miniaci A, Tytherleigh-Strong G. Fixation of unstable osteochondritis dissecans lesions of the knee using arthroscopic autogenous osteochondral grafting (mo-saicplasty). Arthroscopy 2007;23(8):845–51.
41. Murray J, Chitnavis J, Dixon P, et al. Osteochondritis dissecans of the knee; long-term clinical outcome following arthroscopic debridement. Knee 2007;14(2): 94–8.
42. Michael J. Long-term results after operative treatment of osteochondritis disse-cans of the knee joint-30 year results. Int Orthop 2008;32(2):217–21.
43. Gudas R, Simonaityte R, Cekanauskas E, et al. A prospective, randomized clin-ical study of osteochondral autologous transplantation versus microfracture for the treatment of osteochondritis dissecans in the knee joint in children. J Pediatr Orthop 2009;29(7):741–8.
44. Peterson L, Minas T, Brittberg M, et al. Treatment of osteochondritis dissecans of the knee with autologous chondrocyte transplantation. J Bone Joint Surg Am 2003;85(2):17–24.
45. Knutsen G, Drogset J, Engebretsen L, et al. A randomized trial comparing autol-ogous chondrocyte implantation with microfracture. J Bone Joint Surg Am 2007; 89(10):2105–12.
46. Bugbee W, Convery F. Osteochondral allograft transplantation. Clin Sports Med 1999;18(1):67–75.
47. Yamashita F, Sakakida K, Suzo F, et al. The transplantation of an autogenic osteo-chondral fragment for osteochondritis dissecans of the knee. Clin Orthop Relat Res 1985;201:43–50.
48. Lyon R, Nissen C, Liu X, et al. Can fresh osteochondral allografts restore function in juveniles with osteochondritis dissecans of the knee. Clin Orthop Relat Res 2013;471(4):1166–73.
49. Emmerson B, Gortz S, Jamali A, et al. Fresh osteochondral allografting in the treatment of osteochondritis dissecans of the femoral condyle. Am J Sports Med 2007;35(6):907–14.
50. Byrd J, Jones KS. Arthroscopic surgery for isolated capitellar osteochondritis dis-secans in adolescent baseball players: minimum three-year follow-up. Am J Sports Med 2002;30:474–8.
51. Tis JE, Edmonds EW, Bastrom T, et al. Short-term results of arthroscopic treat-ment of osteochondritis dissecans in skeletally immature patients. J Pediatr Or-thop 2012;32(3):226–31.
52. Peterson RK, Savoie FH 3rd, Field LD. Osteochondritis dissecans of the elbow. Instr Course Lect 1999;48:393–8.

53. Stubbs MJ, Field LD, Savoie FH 3rd. Osteochondritis dissecans of the elbow. Clin Sports Med 2001;20:1–9.
54. Miyake J, Kataoka T, Murase T, et al. In-vivo biomechanical analysis of osteochondritis dissecans of the humeral trochlea: a case report. J Pediatr Orthop B 2013;22(4):392–6.
55. Dotzis A, Galissier B, Peyrou P, et al. Osteochondritis dissecans of the radial head: a case report. J Shoulder Elbow Surg 2009;18:e18–21.
56. Zlotolow D, Bae D. Osteochondral autograft transplantation in the elbow. J Hand Surg 2014;39(2):368–72.
57. Kida Y, Morihara T, Hojo T, et al. Prevalence and clinical characteristics of osteochondritis dissecans of the humeral capitellum among adolescent baseball players. Am J Sports Med 2014;42(8):1963–71.
58. Churchill RW, Munoz J, Ahmad CS. Osteochondritis dissecans of the elbow. Curr Rev Musculoskelet Med 2016;9(2):232–9.
59. Lewine EB, Miller PE, Micheli LJ, et al. Early results of drilling and/or microfracture for grade IV osteochondritis dissecans of the capitellum. J Pediatr Orthop 2015; 36(8):803–9.
60. Baker CL 3rd, Romeo AA, Baker CL Jr. Osteochondritis dissecans of the capitellum. Am J Sports Med 2010;38(9):1917–28.
61. Kijowski R, DeSmet AA. Radiography of the elbow for evaluation of patients with osteochondritis dissecans of the capitellum. Skeletal Radiol 2005;34(5):266–71.
62. Satake H, Takahara M, Harada M, et al. Preoperative imaging criteria for unstable osteochondritis dissecans of the capitellum. Clin Orthop Relat Res 2013;471(4): 1137–43.
63. Claessen FM, van den Ende KI, Doornberg JN, et al, Shoulder and Elbow Platform & Science of Variation Group. Osteochondritis dissecans of the humeral capitellum: reliability of four classification systems using radiographs and computed tomography. J Shoulder Elbow Surg 2015;24(10):1613–8.
64. Zbojniewicz AM, Laor T. Imaging of osteochondritis dissecans. Clin Sports Med 2014;33(2):221–50.
65. Jans LB, Ditchfield M, Anna G, et al. MR imaging findings and MR criteria for instability in osteochondritis dissecans of the elbow in children. Eur J Radiol 2012;81(6):1306–10.
66. Takahara M, Mura N, Sasaki J, et al. Classification, treatment, and outcome of osteochondritis dissecans of the humeral capitellum. J Bone Joint Surg Am 2007; 89(6):1205–14.
67. Mihara K, Tsutsui H, Nishinaka N, et al. Nonoperative treatment for osteochondritis dissecans of the capitellum. Am J Sports Med 2009;37(2):298–304.
68. Matsuura T, Kashiwaguchi S, Iwase T, et al. Conservative Treatment for Osteochondrosis of the Humeral Capitellum. Am J Sports Med 2008;36(5):868–72.
69. Shi L, Bae D, Kocher M, et al. Contained versus uncontained lesions in juvenile elbow osteochondritis dissecans. J Pediatr Orthop 2012;32(3):221–5.
70. Mihara K, Suzuki K, Makiuchi D, et al. Surgical treatment for osteochondritis dissecans of the humeral capitellum. J Shoulder Elbow Surg 2010;19:31–7.
71. Kosaka M, Nakase J, Takahashi R, et al. Outcomes and failure factors in surgical treatment for osteochondritis dissecans of the capitellum. J Pediatr Orthop 2013; 33(7):719–24.
72. Jones K, Wiesel B, Sankar W, et al. Arthroscopic management of osteochondritis dissecans of the capitellum: mid-term results in adolescent athletes. J Pediatr Orthop 2010;30(1):8–13.

73. Wulf CA, Stone RM, Giveans MR, et al. Magnetic resonance imaging after arthroscopic microfracture of capitellar osteochondritis dissecans. Am J Sports Med 2012;40:2549–56.
74. Hennrikus W, Miller P, Micheli L, et al. Internal fixation of unstable in situ osteochondritis dissecans lesions of the capitellum. J Pediatr Orthop 2015;35(5): 467–73.
75. Uchida S, Utsunomiya H, Taketa T, et al. Arthroscopic fragment fixation using hydroxyapatite/poly-L-lactate Acid thread pins for treating elbow osteochondritis dissecans. Am J Sports Med 2015;43(5):1057–65.
76. Gancarczyk SM, Makhni EC, Lombardi JM, et al. Arthroscopic articular reconstruction of capitellar osteochondral defects. Am J Sports Med 2015;43(10): 2452–8.
77. Maruyama M, Takahara M, Harada M, et al. Outcomes of an open autologous osteochondral plug graft for capitellar osteochondritis dissecans: time to return to sports. Am J Sports Med 2014;42(8):1963–71.
78. Lyons ML, Werner BC, Gluck JS, et al. Osteochondral autograft plug transfer for treatment of osteochondritis dissecans of the capitellum in adolescent athletes. J Shoulder Elbow Surg 2015;24(7):1098–105.
79. Iwasaki N, Kato H, Ishikawa J, et al. Autologous osteochondral mosaicplasty for osteochondritis dissecans of the elbow in teenage athletes. J Bone Joint Surg Am 2009;91(10):2359–66.
80. Shimada K, Tanaka H, Matsumoto T, et al. Cylindrical costal osteochondral autograft for reconstruction of large defects of the capitellum due to osteochondritis dissecans. J Bone Joint Surg Am 2012;94(11):992–1002.
81. Nishinaka N, Tsutsui H, Yamaguchi K, et al. Costal osteochondral autograft for reconstruction of advanced-stage osteochondritis dissecans of the capitellum. J Shoulder Elbow Surg 2014;23(12):1888–97.
82. Kappis M. Weitese Beitrage zur Traumatisch-mechanischen-Entstehung der Spontanen Knospelablosungen. Dtsch Z Chir 1922;171:13–29.
83. Naumetz VA, Schweigel JF. Osseocartilaginous lesions of the talar dome. J Trauma 1980;20:924–7.
84. Zanon G, DiVico G, Marullo M. Osteochondritis dissecans of the talus. Joints 2014;2(3):115–23.
85. McCullough C, Venugopal V. Osteochondritis dissecans of the talus: the natural history. Clin Orthop Relat Res 1979;144:264–8.
86. Kessler J, Weiss J, Nikizad H, et al. Osteochondritis dissecans of the ankle in children and adolescents: demographics and epidemiology. Am J Sports Med 2014; 42(9):22165–71.
87. DeSmet AA, Fischer D, Burnstein M, et al. Value of MR imaging in staging osteochondral lesions of the talus (osteochondritis dissecans): results in 14 patients. AJR Am J Roentgenol 1990;154:555–8.
88. Letts M, Davidson D, Ahmer A. Osteochondritis dissecans of the talus in children. J Pediatr Orthop 2003;23:617–25.
89. Perumal V, Wall E, Babekir N. Juvenile osteochondritis dissecans of the talus. J Pediatr Orthop 2007;27:821–5.
90. Kramer D, Glotzbecker M, Shore B, et al. Results of surgical management of osteochondritis dissecans of the ankle in the pediatric and adolescent population. J Pediatr Orthop 2015;35(7):725–33.

Osteochondral Autologous Transplantation

Seth L. Sherman, MD[a,b,*], Emil Thyssen, BS[c], Clayton W. Nuelle, MD[a]

KEYWORDS

- Osteochondral autograft transplant • Articular cartilage defect • Techniques
- Outcomes

KEY POINTS

- Osteochondral autologous transplantation (OAT) is a surgical treatment option for active patients with small to medium focal grade III and IV chondral or osteochondral lesions of the knee joint.
- Advantages of OAT include single stage procedure, restoration of hyaline cartilage, and native bone healing.
- Disadvantages of OAT include donor site availability and donor site morbidity, and technical difficulty, often limiting treatment to lesions typically less than 4 cm².
- Strict correction of ligament instability, malalignment, or meniscal deficiency is required to optimize OAT outcomes.
- Clinical studies have demonstrated superior OAT outcomes versus microfracture regarding patient activity level at medium and long-term follow-up.

INTRODUCTION

The optimal treatment of symptomatic focal cartilage defects in the knee joint remains controversial. There are a variety of treatment options available for cartilage repair, including microfracture, cell based repair, and transplantation of autograft or allograft osteochondral units. Osteochondral autologous transplantation (OAT) is a surgical technique that has been developed to treat small or medium

Disclosures: Authors E. Thyssen and C.W. Nuelle report conflict of interest disclosures. S.L. Sherman reports the following disclosures: ACL Study Group: Board or committee member; American Journal of Orthopedics: Editorial or governing board; American Orthopaedic Society for Sports Medicine: Board or committee member; Arthrex: Paid consultant; Research support; Arthroscopy: Editorial or governing board; Arthroscopy Association of North America: Board or committee member; Neotis: Paid consultant; Regeneration Technologies, Inc.: Paid consultant; Vericel: Paid consultant; Zimmer: Research support.
^a Department of Orthopaedic Surgery, University of Missouri, Columbia, MO, USA; ^b Missouri Orthopaedic Institute, 1100 Virginia Avenue, Columbia, MO 65212, USA; ^c School of Medicine, University of Missouri, One Hospital Drive, MA204, Columbia, MO 65212, USA
* Corresponding author.
E-mail address: shermanse@health.missouri.edu

sized symptomatic focal grade III and IV chondral or osteochondral defects in the knee.

The technique was initially described by D'Aubigne in 1945 and has been modified by Outerbridge and others to include both mini-open and arthroscopic transplantation.[1,2] In this procedure, 1 or more autologous osteochondral grafts are harvested from a donor site, typically from a minimally weight bearing zone within the ipsilateral joint, and transplanted to the area of cartilage damage. The primary advantages of this single stage procedure are the rapid bone-to-bone subchondral graft healing and restoration of native type II hyaline cartilage tissue at the articular surface. Limitations of the technique include donor site availability and morbidity, and technical demand with larger lesions requiring multiple osteochondral plugs. Clinical studies have demonstrated return to higher activity levels in OAT patients versus microfracture cohorts, and overall 70% to 90% success rates at 2 to 10 years of follow-up.[3–5] A thorough understanding of the indications, techniques, outcomes, and limitations of OAT is required to optimize surgical results and improve outcomes for our patients.

SURGICAL INDICATIONS AND CONTRAINDICATIONS
Lesion Location

- Initially, OAT was described for cartilage defects in the knee, particularly for lesions of the femoral condyles and the patella.
- At present, OAT may be used for primary treatment of small and medium sized lesions of the femoral condyle, patella, or trochlea, or as a salvage treatment for failed microfracture in these same locations, using a retrograde approach for the tibial plateau.
- When treating focal patella lesions with OAT, care must be taken because there is a mismatch between the thickness of cartilage surface of the donor and recipient sites that leaves an incongruous subchondral bone plate despite a flush articular surface.
- Owing to positive outcomes in these locations, the procedure has been performed for similar defects in the talus, the distal tibia, the proximal and distal humerus, the metacarpal and metatarsal heads, and the femoral head.[6]

Lesion Size

- Symptomatic defects 1 to 2 cm in diameter or 1 to 4 cm^2 in area are indicated for OAT. Treatment of defects less than 1 cm^2 are controversial because they often do not progress or are minimally symptomatic.[7–10]
- It is important to consider the ratio of the defect to the size of the entire knee. For example, a cartilage defect of less than 1 cm^2 may be relevant clinically in a patient with small femoral condyle dimensions.[11]
- Defects greater than 2 cm in diameter or 4 cm^2 in area require multiple grafts, which are limited by donor harvest site availability, and may be better served by other treatment modalities, such as allograft transplantation or autologous chondrocyte implantation.[6,8–10,12]

Lesion Depth

- OAT is indicated for treatment of symptomatic International Cartilage Repair Society grade III or IV defects in a physiologically active patient.[8,9,11] Low-grade lesions may be better treated with observation or chondroplasty for unstable superficial cartilage flaps.

- For small and medium full-thickness osteochondral defects with clear violation of the subchondral bone plate, OAT is the preferred treatment over surface treatments, such as microfracture.
- OAT may also be the preferred treatment over microfracture for lesions with intact subchondral plate, but with substantial underlying subchondral edema.

Patient Selection

- OAT is indicated for the treatment of symptomatic focal chondral or osteochondral knee lesions that have failed conservative treatment options (ie, physical therapy, nonsteroidal antiinflammatory drugs, bracing, injections).
- Patients often present with pain in the location of the lesion, biologic effusions, and major mechanical symptoms.
- Similar to other cartilage treatments, relative and absolute contraindications to autologous osteochondral transplantation include age greater than 50 years, body mass index greater than 40 kg/m^2, knee osteoarthritis with Kellgren-Lawrence grade 2 and above, and a history of knee infections, tumors, or inflammatory arthritis.

Concomitant Procedures

- Similar to other cartilage treatments, strict recognition and correction of knee malalignment, ligament instability, and meniscus deficiency is important to optimize patient outcome with OAT.[6,13,14]
- Ligament stability is critical for cartilage repair. Rotational and translational stability help to normalize contact stress and shear forces, which may damage the transplanted tissue. Ligament repair and reconstruction (ie, anterior cruciate ligament reconstruction) is typically performed at the time of OAT, although these may be performed as staged procedures when necessary.
- Correction of malalignment improves patient outcomes for cartilage restoration and increases graft survival.[11,13,14] This may be performed as a concomitant procedure or as part of the first of staged interventions. For patients with varus malalignment and focal cartilage defect of the medial femoral condyle, an opening wedge high tibial osteotomy is preferred. For patients with valgus malalignment and focal defects of the lateral femoral condyle, a distal femoral osteotomy is recommended. Patellofemoral malalignment is typically corrected with tibial tubercle osteotomy.[11,13,14]
- The menisci are responsible for dispersion of joint forces, appropriate joint contact area, and synovial fluid systems. Therefore, when menisci are deficient, they can lead to severely increased contact forces, osteochondral injury, and joint instability. Additionally, because articular cartilage is nutritionally supplied by synovial fluid, meniscal damage also interrupts the proper synovial fluid dynamics, which are optimal with proper meniscal compression.[11] For these reasons, intact menisci lead to more positive outcomes.

SURGICAL TECHNIQUE
Overview

- There are 2 main types of autologous transplantation procedures: single plug and mosaicplasty.
- The single plug technique is carried out by transplantation of a 6- to 10-mm diameter osteochondral graft/plug that is used to fill the entirety of the cartilage defect.

- The advantage of the single plug technique is the potential to restore the entire surface of cartilage injury with congruent hyaline cartilage. The primary disadvantage is the limited donor site availability and lesions size. This is relevant for donor harvest in small knees and in patients with larger chondral or osteochondral defects.
- Mosaicplasty is carried out by multiple, small diameter osteochondral grafts or plugs producing a mosaic-like structure. The advantage of using multiple, smaller plugs allows potentially easier matching of the surface contour of the defect site and the ability to harvest grafts from multiple donor sites. The disadvantage of multiple plugs includes clefts and space between the grafts, meaning more potential for fibrocartilage ingrowth and less complete hyaline cartilage.[6,15]

Donor Site Harvest

- There are 3 available harvest sites within the knee: the far superior medial and lateral surfaces of the trochlea and the lateral aspect of the intercondylar notch (**Fig. 1**).
- These sites are chosen for their low weight bearing and dimensional properties as well as their curvature, which reduces mismatch to the recipient site.[6,9,16]
- The harvest site with the largest surface area of minimal joint contact pressure, and thus the largest donor site area, is the lateral trochlear flare superior to the sulcus terminalis.
- One review suggests that often the intercondylar notch provides 6-mm grafts, the medial trochlea provides 8-mm grafts, and the lateral trochlea provides 10-mm grafts superior to the sulcus terminalis.[9]

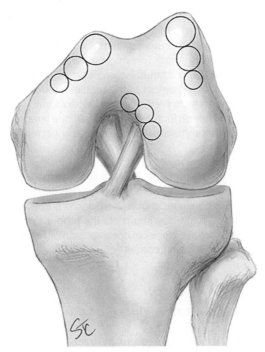

Fig. 1. Potential harvest sites for osteochondral autograft transplantation. (*Courtesy of* University of Missouri, Columbia, MO; with permission.)

- It has been suggested that the donor site should be opposite of the recipient site, such that postoperative pain localization is easier distinguished as donor versus the recipient site (ie, a defect of the medial femoral condyle should be covered by a graft harvested from the lateral trochlea).[9]
- The appropriate sized donor harvester is selected (typically 4–10 mm) and is placed perpendicular to the donor site such that it is flush with the articular cartilage. The perpendicularity is important for donor site integrity and to prohibit stepping at the recipient site after implantation. Extending one of the portals or performing a mini-open arthrotomy may be necessary to ensure appropriate harvester positioning.
- The donor harvester is then gently impacted with a mallet to a depth of 12 to 15 mm. It is important to acquire a minimum of 10 mm to ensure adequate subchondral bone with the harvested graft plug. Once the harvester has reached the appropriate depth, it is turned 180° to cut and disengage the graft from the harvest site. It is important to avoid any toggling of the harvester during this step to avoid graft fracture or creation of incongruity.
- If multiple plugs are to be harvested, separation of each harvest site by 2 mm is preferred to ensure perpendicularity with each harvest. This can be accomplished by flexing or extending the knee and altering the entry point and angles to the knee with the harvester.
- The donor site(s) may be left in situ, with likely fill in with varying amounts of fibrocartilage, grafted with the recipient site bone plug(s), or filled with allograft cancellous bone chips for larger graft sites.
- Alternatively, donor plugs may be taken from the contralateral knee, although this is not the preferred option.

Single Plug Surgical Technique

- The defect is identified and sized using an arthroscopic or mini-open approach (**Fig. 2**). The recipient site is measured for surface area and depth (**Fig. 3**A).
- Through the arthroscopic approach, an 18-gauge spinal needle can be used to assess the available angle of potential graft insertion, because a perpendicular angle is required.

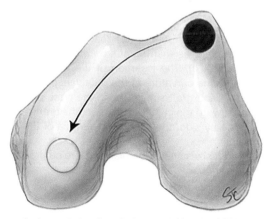

Fig. 2. Single plug technique. Osteochondral autograft transplantation. The donor site is the lateral trochlea above the sulcus and the recipient site is the weight bearing zone of the medial femoral condyle. (*Courtesy of* University of Missouri, Columbia, MO; with permission.)

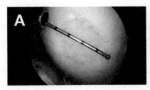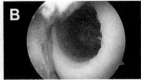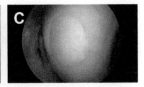

Fig. 3. Case example demonstrating (*A*) focal full-thickness 8 mm condyle defect, (*B*) during recipient preparation, and (*C*) after osteochondral autograft transplantation.

- Mini-arthrotomy is typically used on lesions that are larger and more posterior, because obtaining the proper insertion angle via arthroscopy can be more difficult in these scenarios. A larger arthrotomy may be performed for patellar defects to evert the patella. Arthroscopy may be used for smaller defects in the midportions of the anterior aspect of the femoral condyles.[6,9]
- A recipient harvester is then used to cut and remove the bone to create a socket for the donor graft. The recipient harvester should be positioned perpendicular to the recipient site and impacted to a depth 2 mm less than the depth of the donor graft. A calibrated alignment rod is inserted into the recipient site to determine the depth and the appropriate angle of graft insertion.
- A curette or scalpel is used to create clear, smooth edges of the defect. The recipient site should be adequately prepared to create perpendicular walls circumferentially around the defect. It is important to preserve the walls of the recipient site to ensure a press-fit transplantation and ensure bone-to-bone healing (see **Fig. 3**B).
- A graft delivery tube is then inserted around the graft harvester. A graft pusher is then inserted through the donor harvester such that the graft is flush with the edge of the delivery tube. The delivery tube is then placed perpendicular into the recipient site and the graft is slowly advanced into the socket.
- The graft should be advanced until it is flush with the native surrounding native cartilage, because a mismatch can result in early graft failure.
- A tamp can be used to gently compress the graft until it is flush, but minimal force should be used during graft insertion, because the use of a mallet can result in graft fracture and chondrocyte injury.[17] (see **Fig. 3**C)

Mosaicplasty Surgical Technique

- If a mosaicplasty is to be performed, the same procedure as previously described is the same for as many grafts as may be necessary to fill at least 80% of the defect (**Fig. 4**). The insertion of the grafts should be carried out such that they restore the curvature of the defective condyle.
- The deepest part of each graft should touch the base of the recipient site and should be directed toward the center. If, instead, the grafts are all placed parallel to each other or side by side, the superficial surface of the condyle will be flat, rather than convex.
- In addition, larger graft sizes should be placed more centrally, with smaller grafts placed around the periphery.[9]

OUTCOMES

- Several studies were analyzed to determine success rates of OAT and to compare those outcomes with other procedures for cartilage defects. In summary, Hospital for Special Surgery, International Cartilage Repair Society, International Knee Documentation Committee, Lysholm, Tegner, and modified

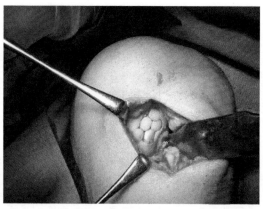

Fig. 4. Miniarthrotomy mosaicplasty on the medial femoral condyle. Five pieces of 6.5-mm grafts were implanted in a flexed knee position. (*From* Hangody L, Vásárhelyi G, Hangody LR, et al. Autologous osteochondral grafting – technique and long-term results. Injury 2008;39(1):S35; with permission.

Cincinnati scores were all higher postoperatively after the OAT procedure. The procedure has consistently shown to improve outcomes, regardless of scoring system.

- **Table 1** provides outcomes of OAT for the knee joint and compares OAT with other cartilage procedures for the treatment of focal chondral and osteochondral defects.[14,18–23]

LIMITATIONS AND COMPLICATIONS

- Donor site availability is a concern, particularly in the setting of smaller knees or for the treatment of larger lesions. Given the harvest requirements from areas of low stress, similar convexity to the defect, and compliant thickness, there are only limited useable areas.[6,9,16] For larger lesions (<4 cm^2), alternative cartilage restoration techniques such as osteochondral allograft or autologous chondrocyte implantation may be preferred.
- Donor site morbidity is a potential complication. Gudas and colleagues[16] demonstrated that 10-mm grafts produced more donor site morbidity and they favor the use of 8-mm grafts. Poor harvesting technique or minimal spacing between donor sites may lead to increased donor site morbidity.[4,6,13]
- Donor recipient graft incongruity is a potential complication of this technique. Harvesting a cylinder from a site that has curvature that is nonuniform with the site of the defect can lead to poor outcomes. In a study of osteochondral grafting in sheep models, there were 3 groups for graft surface: congruent, countersunk 1 mm, and countersunk 2 mm. The study found that the defects filled with grafts that were congruent or countersunk no more than 1 mm had preserved, hypertrophied hyaline cartilage. Grafts that were more than 1 mm countersunk or left proud have shown higher rates of resorption, necrosis, and worse outcomes.[24,25]
- Mosaicplasty is technically demanding for larger lesions. The potential for incongruous surface, gapping between plugs with fibrocartilaginous fill, and donor site morbidity make the use of OAT with more than 2 or 3 plugs less desirable than using other cartilage restoration techniques.

Table 1
Outcomes of OAT versus other procedures for articular cartilage defects

Procedure	Study Design	Level of Evidence	Defect Size	Study Duration	Results	Conclusions
OAT vs MF; Gudas et al,[18] 2005	Prospective RCT n = 60 Average age 24.3 ± 6.8 y Lesions of MFC, LFC	I	Mean 2.80 ± 0.65 cm²	12, 24, and 36 mo	HSS scores were significantly higher (P <.1) in the OAT group (91.1 ± 4.1) compared with MF (80.6 ± 4.6). ICRS scores were also significantly higher (P <.001) in the OAT group (89 ± 4) compared with MF (75 ± 4).	OAT has significantly better outcomes compared with MF in well-trained, high-demand athletes
OAT vs MF; Gudas et al,[19] 2012	Prospective RCT n = 60 Average age 24.3 ± 6.8 y Lesions of condyles	I	Mean 2.80 ± 0.65 cm²	124.8 mo (range, 86–132)	ICRS scores were significantly higher (P <.001) in both groups after the procedure. At 10 y follow-up, the OAT group had a 14% failure rate compared with a 38% failure rate in the MF group.	Athletes <30 y had better outcomes with both procedures than athletes >30 y (P = .008)
OAT vs MF vs debridement; Gudas et al,[16] 2013	Prospective RCT n = 102 Average age 34.1 y Lesions of MFC	II	Mean 2.6 cm²	36.1 mo (range, 34–37)	IKDC scores were significantly higher (P <.005) in all groups at 3 y follow-up. The OAT group IKDC scores were significantly higher than the MF group (P <.024) and D group (P <.018).	When an articular cartilage defect is present during ACL reconstruction, IKDC scores are significantly better for OAT vs MF vs debridement at 3-y follow-up. Anterior knee stability was not significantly affected by any method.

OAT vs MF vs ACI; Lim et al,[20] 2012	Prospective RCT n = 70 Average age 32.9 y Lesions of MFC, LFC	=	Mean 2.74 cm^2	80.4 mo (range, 42–126)	Lysholm, Tegner, and HSS scores all improved postoperatively in each group. There was no difference among the groups in postoperative scores.	OAT, MF, and ACI are all appropriate treatment options for articular cartilage defects because they all improve outcomes. However, no single procedure was significantly superior to any other.
OAT vs ACI-P; Horas et al,[21] 2003	Prospective RCT n = 40 Average Age 33.4 y Lesions of MFC, LFC	=	Mean 3.75 cm^2	6, 12, and 24 mo	Lysholm scores were significantly higher at 6 (P <.015), 12 (P <.001), and 24 mo (P <.012) in the OAT group (74 ± 6) vs the ACI-P group (67 ± 8). Meyers and Tegner scores were not different between the groups. Histologic evaluation showed gap filling with hyaline cartilage in the OAT group and fibrocartilage in the ACI-P group.	Both OAT and ACI-P produce positive outcomes in patients. However, both the Lysholm scores and the histologic evaluation of OAT was more positive than the ACI-P in these patients.

(continued on next page)

Table 1
(continued)

Procedure	Study Design	Level of Evidence	Defect Size	Study Duration	Results	Conclusions
OAT vs ACI; Bentley et al,[22] 2003	Prospective RCT n = 100 Average age 31.3 y Lesions of MFC, LFC, trochlea, patella, tibial plateau	I	Mean 4.66 cm^2	19 mo (range, 12–26)	A modified Cincinnati score > 55 was higher ($P = .27$) in the ACI group (88%) than the OAT group (69%). The percent of patients with a CRA of 8–12 was significantly higher ($P <.01$) in the ACI group (82%) than the OAT group (34%) on arthroscopy.	ACI produced significantly superior cartilage on arthroscopy compared with OAT for repairing articular defects of the knee. Clinical outcomes were also higher in the ACI group than the OAT group, although the finding was not statistically significant.
OAT vs ACI; Bentley et al,[23] 2012	10 y follow-up to prospective RCT study n = 100 Average age 31.3 y Lesions of MFC, LFC, trochlea, patella, tibial plateau	I	Mean 4.66 cm^2	Minimum 10 y	A modified Cincinnati score >55 was significantly higher ($P = .02$) in the ACI group than the OAT group. Failure at 10 y was significantly higher ($P <.001$) in the OAT group (55%) compared with ACI (17%).	At a 10-y follow-up, ACI produces significantly higher clinical outcomes than OAT, and OAT was significantly more likely to fail compared with ACI.

Abbreviations: ACI, autologous chondrocyte implantation; ACI-P, autologous chondrocyte implantation – periosteal; ACL, anterior cruciate ligament; CRA, cartilage repair assessment; D, debridement; HSS, Hospital for Special Surgery; ICRS, International Cartilage Repair Society; IKDC, International Knee Documentation Committee; LFC, lateral femoral condyle; MF, microfracture; MFC, medial femoral condyle; OAT, osteochondral autograft transplantation; RCT, randomized, controlled trial.

- Performing OAT without recognizing and treating concomitant pathology increases the risk of early failure. The rates of failure increase with uncorrected ligament instability, malalignment, or untreated meniscal deficiency.

SUMMARY

Osteochondral autograft transplantation is a surgical treatment option for active patients with small or medium sized symptomatic, grade III and IV osteochondral defects of the knee joint. Primary advantages of this minimally invasive technique include single stage cartilage repair with restoration of mature hyaline cartilage and rapid native bone-to-bone subchondral healing. Disadvantages include potential donor site morbidity, limited donor site availability, and the technical demands of the procedure. Clinical studies have demonstrated superior outcomes of OAT versus microfracture with regard to patient activity levels at final follow-up. Similar to other cartilage restoration techniques, strict correction of ligament instability, malalignment, and meniscal deficiency is required to improve patient outcome. Overall, OAT is a valuable tool in the arsenal to treat chondral or osteochondral knee lesions.

ACKNOWLEDGMENT

The authors thank Stacy T. Cheavens, MS, Certified Medical Illustrator, University of Missouri, for creating figure illustrations.

REFERENCES

1. Outerbridge HK, Outerbridge AR, Outerbridge RE. The use of a lateral patellar autologous graft for the repair of a large osteochondral defect in the knee. J Bone Joint Surg Am 1995;77:65–72.
2. Barber FA, Chow JC. Arthroscopic osteochondral transplantation: histologic results. Arthroscopy 2001;17:832–5.
3. Barber FA, Chow JC. Arthroscopic chondral osseous autograft transplantation for femoral defects. Arthroscopy 2006;22:10–6.
4. Krych AJ, Harnly HW, Rodeo SA, et al. Activity levels are higher after osteochondral autograft transfer mosaicplasty than after microfracture for articular cartilage defects of the knee; a retrospective comparative study. J Bone Joint Surg Am 2012;94:971–8.
5. Marcacci M, Kon E, Delcogliano M, et al. Arthroscopic autologous osteochondral grafting for cartilage defects of the knee: prospective study results at a minimum 7-year follow-up. Am J Sports Med 2007;35:2014–21.
6. Hangody L, Vasarhelyi G, Hangody LR, et al. Autologous osteochondral grafting-technique and long-term results. Injury 2008;39(suppl 1):S32–9.
7. Bhosale AM, Richardson JB. Articular cartilage: structure, injuries and review of management. Br Med Bull 2008;87:77–95.
8. Harris JD, Siston RA, Pan X, et al. Autologous chondrocyte implantation: a systematic review. J Bone Joint Surg Am 2010;92:2220–33.
9. Robert H. Chondral repair of the knee joint using mosaicplasty. Orthop Traumatol Surg Res 2011;97:418–29.
10. Kodali P, Parker RD. Articular cartilage restoration: the shape of things to come. Semin Arthroplasty 2010;21:72–6.
11. Mall NA, Harris JD, Cole BJ. Clinical evaluation and preoperative planning of articular cartilage lesions of the knee. J Am Acad Orthop Surg 2015;23:633–40.

12. Brucker PU, Paul J, Imhoff AB. Mega-OATS. In: Brittberg M, Gersoff WK, editors. Cartilage surgery – an operative manual. Philadelphia: Elsevier Saunders; 2011. p. 83–94.

13. Moran CJ, Pascual-Garrido C, Chubinskaya S, et al. Restoration of articular cartilage. J Bone Joint Surg Am 2014;96:336–44.

14. Sherman SL, Garrity J, Bauer K, et al. Fresh osteochondral allograft transplantation for the knee: current concepts. J Am Acad Orthop Surg 2014;22:121–33.

15. Hangody L, Dobos J, Balo E, et al. Clinical experiences with autologous osteochondral mosaicplasty in an athletic population: a 17-year prospective multicenter study. Am J Sports Med 2010;38:1125–33.

16. Gudas R, Gudaitè A, Mickevičius T, et al. Comparison of osteochondral autologous transplantation, microfracture, or debridement techniques in articular cartilage lesions associated with anterior cruciate ligament injury: a prospective study with a 3-year follow-up. Arthroscopy 2013;29:89–97.

17. Sgaglione NA, Chen E, Bert JM, et al. Current strategies for nonsurgical, arthroscopic, and minimally invasive surgical treatment of knee cartilage pathology. Instr Course Lect 2010;59:157–80.

18. Gudas R, Kalesinskas RJ, Kimtys V, et al. A prospective randomized clinical study of mosaic osteochondral autologous transplantation versus microfracture for the treatment of osteochondral defects in the knee joint in young athletes. Arthroscopy 2005;21:1066–75.

19. Gudas R, Gudaite A, Pocius A, et al. Ten-year follow-up of a prospective, randomized clinical study of mosaic osteochondral autologous transplantation versus micro- fracture for the treatment of osteochondral defects in the knee joint of athletes. Am J Sports Med 2012;40:2499–508.

20. Lim HC, Bae JH, Song SH, et al. Current treatments of isolated articular cartilage lesions of the knee achieve similar outcomes. Clin Orthop Relat Res 2012;470:2261–7.

21. Horas U, Pelinkovic D, Herr G, et al. Autologous chondrocyte implantation and osteochondral cylinder transplantation in cartilage repair of the knee joint. A prospective, comparative trial. J Bone Joint Surg Am 2003;85A:185–92.

22. Bentley G, Biant LC, Carrington RW, et al. A prospective, randomised comparison of autologous chondrocyte implantation versus mosaicplasty for osteochondral defects in the knee. J Bone Joint Surg Br 2003;85:223–30.

23. Bentley G, Biant LC, Vijayan S, et al. Minimum ten-year results of a prospective randomised study of autologous chondrocyte implantation versus mosaicplasty for symptomatic articular cartilage lesions of the knee. J Bone Joint Surg Br 2012;94:504–9.

24. Huang FS, Simonean PT, Norman AG, et al. Effects of small incongruities in a sheep model of osteochondral grafting. Am J Sports Med 2004;32:1842–8.

25. Patil S, Tapasvi SR. Osteochondral autografts. Curr Rev Musculoskelet Med 2015;8:423–8.

Microfracture and Microfracture Plus

Jay C. Albright, MD*, Ariel Kiyomi Daoud, BA

KEYWORDS

- Osteochondral defects • Osteochondral allografts • Articular cartilage
- Hyaline cartilage • Microfracture

KEY POINTS

- Review indications for microfracture with or without augmentation.
- Review outcomes of microfracture with or without augmentation.
- Review surgical technical considerations.

INTRODUCTION

Marrow stimulation of the bone bed of a cartilage lesion is a mainstay of cartilage defect surgery. However, with limited long-term success compared with chondroplasty/debridement of lesions, attempts to improve this treatment continue to evolve. The goal of any technique is to restore the cartilage surface to as-close-to the native state as possible and to return the joint to its natural biomechanics and biology. Cost-effectiveness continues to be of concern for health institutions and patients. The ability to care for patients in the most cost-effective manner must also be considered. With the limited biological environment in which cartilage resides, attempts at repair are further constrained. This limitation results in fibrocartilage healing of the defect, which is inferior to healing by hyaline cartilage. Enhancing this environment to create a more hospitable area for healing with as-close-to native cartilage as possible in a single-stage fashion would be ideal for the treatment of chondral injuries. The authors review the technical aspects of microfracture with or without augmentation and the outcomes of healing with these techniques.

BACKGROUND

Marrow stimulation with the Pridie procedure (microfracture) or abrasion arthroplasty has been used as a technique for the attempted healing of chondral injury since Insall[1] reported on the Pridie procedure in 1974. In the short-term, small lesions seem to do well; however, microfracture has had limited success in larger lesions.[2–6]

Disclosure Statement: The lead author, J.C. Albright, participates in a national outcomes registry study hosted by Arthrex Inc and is nominally reimbursed on a per-patient basis for use of BioCartilage in knee arthroscopy.
Department of Orthopedics, Children's Hospital Colorado, University of Colorado, 13123 East 16th Avenue, B060, Aurora, CO 80045, USA
* Corresponding author.
E-mail address: jay.albright@childrenscolorado.org

Clin Sports Med 36 (2017) 501–507
http://dx.doi.org/10.1016/j.csm.2017.02.012
0278-5919/17/© 2017 Elsevier Inc. All rights reserved.

sportsmed.theclinics.com

Meta-analyses confirm that results for larger lesions deteriorate over time (after 2 years) and that after 5 years any size lesion treatment can be expected to fail.[6–8] In pediatric patients with osteochondritis dissecans, there is no difference in outcomes with or without microfracture added to simple debridement.[9] In fact, more than 90% of the time, fibrocartilage will form in a chondral defect without marrow stimulation if the damaged area is unloaded by correcting malalignment.[10–12]

Augmentation with a scaffold follows the rationale that the goal of cartilage injury treatment is to provide a viable cost-effective long-term solution for patients in a single surgery. Other current techniques for cartilage restoration or regeneration are nonoptimal because of the morbidity of a donor site (osteochondral autografts), requirement of a second procedure (autologous chondrocyte implantation [ACI]), need for donor availability (allograft sources), limited shelf life, or are limited in exploitation of biological regeneration sources (Cartilage Autograft Implantation System, DePuy Mitek, Inc, Norwood, MA; or DeNovo, Zimmer, Warsaw, IN).[13–20] Although microfracture allows for mesenchymal cells to access the cartilage defect, it forms fibrocartilage without significant return of the normal biomechanics of hyaline cartilage.[21] More recent attempts are being made to approach a reliable single-stage surgery that can regenerate a durable hyaline cartilage and will stand up long-term. In 2013, Irion and Flanigan[22] described scaffold-based technologies around the world that were not available for public use and had promising but short-term successes. These scaffolds generally fall into 4 main classes: (1) synthetic, (2) protein based, (3) carbohydrate based, or (4) a combination.[22] Kon and colleagues[23] reviewed the literature that compared use of scaffoldings with and without autologous cells and found no absolute significant difference in success rates. These findings further support a single-stage surgery. Chawla and colleagues[24] reviewed the literature for pediatric patients showing that, with greater than 3 cm^2 lesions, there was improvement in patient outcomes using osteochondral autograft transplantation, or one of the 3 generations of ACI, although microfracture also improved outcomes up to 4 years postoperatively particularly in smaller lesions.[25–37] Although more human and long-term studies of all these scaffolds are needed, BioCartilage (Arthrex Inc, Naples, FL) has been shown to produce the desired result of hyaline cartilage regeneration in animal models. Combined with its relative low cost compared with other commercially available materials and promising initial results, it is a viable option for first-line surgical treatment of these injuries.[13]

At present, there is a marked lack of literature considering the short- or long-term clinical outcomes of microfracture alone versus microfracture with the addition of a scaffold. Xing and colleagues[21] (2013) randomized 66 rabbits into a microfracture group and a microfracture plus osteochondral paste (experimental) group and studied regenerated tissues at 4, 8, and 12 weeks postoperatively. The experimental group boasted majority hyaline-like regenerate tissue, whereas microfracture alone was fibrocartilagelike tissue mostly at 12 weeks. The glycosaminoglycan content was significantly increased in the experiment group at all 3 time points and collagen gene expression higher at 12 weeks, indicating greater-quality tissue healing. These short-term animal model results encourage long-term improved outcomes for use of microfracture plus scaffolding in humans.

INDICATIONS FOR MICROFRACTURE ALONE OR WITH THE ADDITION OF A SINGLE-STAGE SCAFFOLDING

Based on the aforementioned literature, there is no true consensus on indications for optimal surgical treatments per patient. Thus, the general approach to be adopted for osteochondral or chondral injuries involves patient-shared decision-making. When direct repair is not possible for small lesions, less than 1 cm^2, debridement with or without microfracture is a reasonable alternative. For lesions measuring 1 to 2 cm^2 and larger, microfracture with single-stage scaffolding is a reasonable and promising first line of defense, though further research needs to be done for definitive prescription. Of the products available in the United States, BioCartilage is relatively inexpensive (less than $2000), and its 5-year shelf life makes storage practical. This scaffolding has promise to produce a viable cartilage regenerative tissue in a single-stage procedure.[13]

TECHNICAL CONSIDERATIONS

After patients have been indicated for surgical intervention, it is most important that the scaffolding considered for use should be available to the surgeon and his or her team.[13] BioCartilage is suitable for staging for use, as its shelf life is years compared with particulate allograft cartilage, such as DeNovo, which has a shelf life of a few weeks. If on surgical inspection, the lesion is smaller than expected, BioCartilage circumvents concern for wasting products or money if the defect does not warrant that treatment.

A thorough arthroscopic evaluation is necessary for the surgeon to confirm all other injuries and pathologic conditions are addressed as needed and that the lesion is or is not reparable. Once the size of the lesion is ascertained the surgeon can also determine if the microfracture and/or scaffolding implantation can be done arthroscopically or if an arthrotomy is required to complete all necessary procedures.

Meticulous preparation of the defect is necessary to remove poor quality tissue at the bone level and to remove damaged, flapped or fibrillated cartilage at the rim. Vertical walls of as–healthy-as-possible cartilage are desired. Accordingly, care must be taken during preparation of the lesion. Bone preparation also depends on chronicity of the lesion. Acute injuries that are not reparable may already traverse through the calcified cartilage layer and thus minimal microfracture or bone penetration is necessary except to remove poorly healing tissue. Chronic lesions, as are typical in osteochondritis dissecans, will likely involve the calcified cartilage layer; however, chronic lesions will also have a thickened rind of subchondral bone that prevents the cancellous blood supply from reaching the lesion. In this situation, penetration of the rind is necessary to obtain extravasation of mesenchymal stem cells into the lesion for microfracture or the addition of Biocartilage to produce healing tissue as desired. Microfracture is then carried out, placing bone tunnels that penetrate the subchondral bone deep enough to reach the marrow elements at 2-mm intervals (**Fig. 1**).

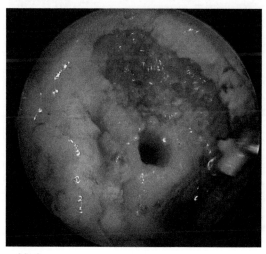

Fig. 1. Microfractured lesion.

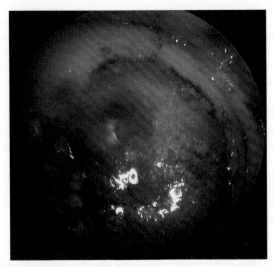

Fig. 2. Implanted BioCartilage.

If the lesion is of critical size that microfracture alone is not likely to result in good long-term outcomes, then BioCartilage is added to the defect. The acellular micronized cartilage matrix is mixed thoroughly with platelet-rich plasma (PRP) in a delivery syringe. A total of 1 mL of PRP is typically enough to obtain the consistency necessary to allow for injection of the mixture into the lesion without too much fluidity. The mixture is then injected into the lesion, filling the lesion until it is 1 mm below the surrounding rim of cartilage. Overfilling or too much fluidity may result in extrusion of a portion or all of the mixed BioCartilage when it is placed through a range of motion and contacts the opposite side of the joint (**Fig. 2**). The BioCartilage mixture is smoothed to make certain the defect is filled evenly, and fibrin glue is used to seal the mixture into the lesion in a drop-by-drop fashion. Too much fibrin glue will leak throughout the joint and create adhesion to soft tissue, which may also dislodge the construct from the defect (**Fig. 3**). The glue

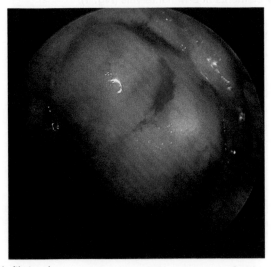

Fig. 3. Sealed with fibrin glue.

is allowed to sit for 5 minutes of dry time; excess glue is carefully removed, and then the joint is placed through a range of motion to ensure the lesion is secured without dislodgement of the construct. If attempting to perform this implantation arthroscopically without arthrotomy, a dry scope view with a maximally dry lesion is necessary. This dehydration is particularly important while the fibrin glue is placed and congealing. The wounds are then closed in standard fashion.

REHABILITATION

With or without augmentation, a joint should be treated like a microfracture postoperatively. This treatment includes touch-down weight bearing for 6 to 8 weeks in femoral or tibial lesions and weight bearing as tolerated for patellar/trochlear lesions while protected in a straight leg brace. Forty-eight to 72 hours of immobilization is preferred before range of motion with consideration of a continuous passive motion device.

REFERENCES

1. Insall J. The Pridie debridement operation for osteoarthritis of the knee. Clin Orthop Relat Res 1974;101:61–7.
2. Bert JM, Maschka K. The arthroscopic treatment of unicompartmental gonarthrosis: a five-year follow-up study of abrasion arthroplasty plus arthroscopic debridement and arthroscopic debridement alone. Arthroscopy 1989;5:25–32.
3. Curl WW, Krome J, Gordon ES, et al. Cartilage injuries: a review of 31,516 knee arthroscopies. Arthroscopy 1997;13:456–60.
4. Hjelle K, Solheim E, Strand T, et al. Articular cartilage defects in 1,000 knee arthroscopies. Arthroscopy 2002;18:730–4.
5. Ciccotti MC, Kraeutler MJ, Austin L, et al. The incidence of articular cartilage changes in the knee joint with increasing age in patients undergoing arthroscopy for meniscal pathology. Arthroscopy 2012;28:1437–44.
6. Mithoefer C, McAdams T, Williams RJ, et al. Current concepts: clinical efficacy of the microfracture technique for articular cartilage repair in the knee: an evidence-based systematic analysis. Am J Sports Med 2009;37:2053–63.
7. Kon E, Filardo G, Berruto M, et al. Articular cartilage treatment in high-level male soccer players: a prospective comparative study of arthroscopic second generation autologous chondrocyte implantation versus microfracture. Am J Sports Med 2011;39:2549–57.
8. Goyal D, Keyhani S, Lee EH, et al. Evidence-based status of microfracture technique: a systematic review of level I and II studies. Arthroscopy 2013;29:1579–88.
9. Gudas R, Gudaitė A, Mickevičius T, et al. Comparison of osteochondral autologous transplantation, microfracture, or debridement techniques in articular cartilage lesions associated with anterior cruciate ligament injury: a prospective study with a 3-year follow-up. Arthroscopy 2013;29:89–91.
10. Jung W-H, Takeuchi R, Chun C-W, et al. Second-look arthroscopic assessment of cartilage regeneration after medial opening-wedge high tibial osteotomy. Arthroscopy 2014;30:72–9.
11. Schultz W, Göbel D. Articular cartilage regeneration of the knee joint after proximal tibial valgus osteotomy: a prospective study of different intra- and extra-articular operative techniques. Knee Surg Sports Traumatol Arthrosc 1999;7: 29–36.
12. Hinterwimmer S, Jaeger A, von Eisenhart-Rothe R, et al. Cartilage morphology after high tibial osteotomy for varus gonarthrosis. Arthroscopy 2012;28:e361–2 [suppl, abstr].

13. Abrams G, Mall N, Fortier L, et al. Biocartilage: background and operative technique. Oper Tech Sports Med 2013;21:116–24.

14. Homminga GN, Bulstra SK, Bouwmeester PS, et al. Perichondral grafting for cartilage lesions of the knee. J Bone Joint Surg Br 1990;72:1003–7.

15. Lubiatowski P, Manikowski W, Romanowski L, et al. The experimental reconstruction of articular cartilage using autogenous periosteal and perichondreal implants. Ortop Traumatol Rehabil 2001;3:194–9.

16. Brittberg M, Lindahl A, Nilsson A, et al. Treatment of deep cartilage defects in the knee with autologous chondrocyte transplantation. N Engl J Med 1994;331:889–95.

17. Vanlauwe J, Saris DB, Victor J, et al. Five-year outcome of characterized chondrocyte implantation versus microfracture for symptomatic cartilage defects of the knee: early treatment matters. Am J Sports Med 2011;39:2566–74.

18. Hangody L, Fules P. Autologous osteochondral mosaicplasty for the treatment of full-thickness defects of weight-bearing joints: ten years of experimental and clinical experience. J Bone Joint Surg Am 2003;85A:25–32.

19. Krych AJ, Robertson CM, Williams RJ 3rd. Return to athletic activity after osteochondral allograft transplantation in the knee. Am J Sports Med 2012;40:1053–9.

20. Gille J, Schuseil E, Wimmer J, et al. Mid-term results of autologous matrix-induced chondrogenesis for treatment of focal cartilage defects in the knee. Knee Surg Sports Traumatol Arthrosc 2010;18:1456–64.

21. Xing L, Jiang Y, Gui J, et al. Microfracture combined with osteochondral paste implantation was more effective than microfracture alone for full-thickness cartilage repair. Knee Surg Sports Traumatol Arthrosc 2013;21(8):1770–6.

22. Irion VH, Flanigan DC. New and emerging techniques in cartilage repair: other scaffold-based cartilage treatment options. Oper Tech Sports Med 2013;21:125–37.

23. Kon E, Roffi A, Filardo G, et al. Scaffold-based cartilage treatments: with or without cells? A systematic review of preclinical and clinical evidence. Arthroscopy 2015;31(4):767–75.

24. Chawla A, Twycross-Lewis R, Maffulli N. Microfracture produces inferior outcomes to other cartilage repair techniques in chondral injuries in the paediatric knee. Br Med Bull 2015;116:93–103.

25. Mithöfer K, Minas T, Peterson L, et al. Functional outcome of knee articular cartilage repair in adolescent athletes. Am J Sports Med 2005;33:1147–53.

26. Micheli LJ, Moseley JB, Anderson AF, et al. Articular cartilage defects of the distal femur in children and adolescents: treatment with autologous chondrocyte implantation. J Pediatr Orthop 2006;26:455–60.

27. Teo BJX, Buhary K, Tai B, et al. Cell-based therapy improves function in adolescents and young adults with patellar osteochondritis dissecans. Clin Orthop Relat Res 2013;471:1152–8.

28. Macmull S, Parratt MT, Bentley G, et al. Autologous chondrocyte implantation in the adolescent knee. Am J Sports Med 2011;39:1723–30.

29. Lyon R, Nissen C, Liu XC, et al. Can fresh osteochondral allografts restore function in juveniles with osteochondritis dissecans of the knee? Clin Orthop Relat Res 2013;471:1166–73.

30. Dai XS, Cai YZ. Matrix-induced autologous chondrocyte implantation addressing focal chondral defect in adolescent knee. Chin Med J 2012;125:4130–3.

31. Gudas R, Simonaityte R, Cekanauskas E, et al. A prospective, randomized clinical study of osteochondral autologous transplantation versus microfracture for

the treatment of osteochondritis dissecans in the knee joint in children. J Pediatr Orthop 2009;29:741–8.

32. Miura K, Ishibashi Y, Tsuda E, et al. Results of arthroscopic fixation of osteochondritis dissecans lesion of the knee with cylindrical autogenous osteochondral plugs. Am J Sports Med 2007;35:216–22.

33. Murphy RT, Pennock AT, Bugbee WD. Osteochondral allograft transplantation of the knee in the pediatric and adolescent population. Am J Sports Med 2014;42: 635–40.

34. Salzmann GM, Sah BR, Schmal H, et al. Microfracture for treatment of knee cartilage defects in children and adolescents. Pediatr Rep 2012;4:e21.

35. Sasaki K, Matsumoto T, Matsushita T, et al. Osteochondral autograft transplantation for juvenile osteochondritis dissecans of the knee: a series of twelve cases. Int Orthop 2012;36:2243–8.

36. Behrens P, Bitter T, Kurz B, et al. Matrix-associated autologous chondrocyte transplantation/implantation (MACT/MACI)—5-year follow-up. Knee 2006;13: 194–202.

37. Steadman JR, Briggs KK, Matheny LM, et al. Outcomes following microfracture of full-thickness articular cartilage. J Knee Surg 2014;28:145–50.

Allografts
Osteochondral, Shell, and Paste

Frank B. Wydra, MD, Philip J. York, MD, Armando F. Vidal, MD*

KEYWORDS

- Osteochondral defects • Osteochondral allografts • Articular cartilage
- Hyaline cartilage • Storage • Procurement • Bacterial transmission

KEY POINTS

- There is an increasing need for articular cartilage restoration procedures, especially in younger active individuals; persistent osteochondral defects can lead to early and rapid degenerative changes.
- Techniques such as microfracture and autologous chondrocyte implantation provide reasonable outcomes for smaller defects without bone loss.
- However, these techniques have very limited effectiveness for lesions greater than 4 cm^2 and lesions with significant bony involvement.
- Ostochondral allografts provide a reasonable option for lesions this large and lesions with subchondral bone loss.
- Emerging options such as cryopreserved viable osteochondral allografts and particulated articular grafts provide different approaches to difficult cartilage defects.

INTRODUCTION

Over the years, the principles and techniques of treatment for chondral injuries continue to evolve. The goals of treatment are to reestablish the natural biomechanics and native biology of a joint while allowing the patient early return to their preinjury state with no long-term sequela. Although several options exist for the treatment of articular cartilage damage, no current option has been able to meet each of these goals. The challenge is present because articular cartilage does not have the inherent ability to regenerate. Many current treatment options result in healing via fibrocartilage, which is biologically and biomechanically inferior to native articular hyaline cartilage. Osteochondral allografts (OCAs), however, are an exception to this. The major strength of OCAs lies in their potential to heal with intact hyaline cartilage. This article discusses the use of allografts, in their various forms, for the use of articular cartilage

Disclosure Statement: The authors of this article have nothing to disclose.
Department of Orthopedics, University of Colorado School of Medicine, 12631 East 17th Avenue, Room 4501 B202, Aurora, CO 80045, USA
* Corresponding author. 12631 East 17th Avenue, Room 4501 B202, Aurora, CO 80045.
E-mail address: armando.vidal@ucdenver.edu

damage. We review the current procurement, screening, storage, and handling process, potential infections, outcomes, as well as how the grafts are used for cartilage damage.

BACKGROUND

The use of OCAs was first reported in the early 1900s and has a growing interest in treatment for articular defects.[1] In 2006, the American Orthopaedic Society for Sports Medicine conducted a survey asking orthopaedic surgeons from around the United States about their usage and concerns of allografts.[2,3] Of the 365 participants,86% endorsed using allografts in some form in their practice. The same participants raised concerns regarding safety, tissue integrity after storage, potential for transmission of infection, and the degree of incorporation of transplanted tissue. Many respondents did not understand or know the intricacies of the screening and storage process. To safely and effectively use allografts, it is essential for the orthopedic surgeon to recognize the current standards of tissue banking, risks and benefits related to the use of allografts, and common indications for safe use in clinical practice.

OSTEOCHONDRAL ALLOGRAFT USES

Damage to articular cartilage comes in various forms, patterns, and sizes. Large osteochondral defects pose a significant dilemma for the orthopaedic surgeon, particularly in young, active patients, who most would like to delay any form of arthroplasty procedure. Options such as microfracture and autologous cartilage implantation have been reasonable options for smaller defects (<2 cm^2) that are well-contained. There is some gray area for lesions between 2 and 4 cm^2, although there is a general consensus that microfracture is inferior to other options such as autologous chondrocyte implantation or OCAs.[4] OCAs are ideally suited for larger (>4 cm^2) lesions, uncontained lesions, multiple defects, lesions with significant subchondral bone loss such as osteochondritis dissecans, and in revision circumstances as they provide a large graft (**Fig. 1**). As with any articular cartilage procedure, the decision for surgery needs to occur in the context of associated limb alignment, stability and meniscal status. Despite their versatility and limitless size, OCAs are not indicated for the treatment of generalized osteoarthritis. Allografts can be matched and templated based on the size and anatomy of the donor before surgery.

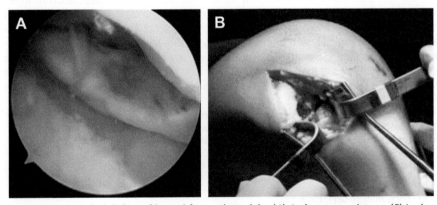

Fig. 1. Osteochondral defect of lateral femoral condyle. (*A*) Arthroscopy picture. (*B*) Lesions directly visualized after arthrotomy.

SCREENING, PROCUREMENT, AND STORAGE PROCESSES

The American Association of Tissue Banks (AATB) is responsible for establishing and enforcing the current standards of more than 100 accredited tissue banks. These tissue banks are responsible for harvesting tissue from nearly 30,000 donors annually and account for approximately 90% of all musculoskeletal allografts used in the United States. Although it is not required that all tissue banks are accredited by the AATB, they are required to register with the Food and Drug Administration (FDA). This registration entitles the FDA to make unannounced inspections of any facility. In 2005, the FDA implemented the Current Good Tissue Practices, which established regulations that all tissue banks are required to follow to help prevent the transmission of communicable diseases. The FDA released an updated proposal in 2009 detailing safe practices and regulations spanning from environmental control to equipment specifics.[5]

The safety and screening process for donor tissue begins at the time of procurement. The first step of screening includes an in-depth analysis of a potential donor's medical and social history. This may be obtained from previous available medical records, talking to family members, and any other health care resources. If prior blood donations or autopsy information is available, that information is scrutinized for previous infections. Ideally, this is accomplished early, because there is a time-sensitive relationship of intestinal migration of bacteria to surrounding tissue. This is a potential source for contamination of donor tissues; therefore, procurement must take place within 24 hours post mortem.[6]

Nucleic acid testing (NAT) of donors is required by both the AATB and FDA, which allows for screening of a variety of viruses that would exclude individuals from being potential donors. The introduction of NAT has significantly reduced viral transmission of hepatitis B virus, hepatitis C virus, human immunodeficiency virus (HIV), *Treponema pallidum*, and human transmissible spongiform encephalopathies.[7] The donors also undergo routine preprocessing swabs for bacterial and fungal cultures; however, the sensitivities of these cultures ranges from 78% to 92%, raising concern for their clinical relevance.[8]

After the aforementioned screening and testing processes, allograft tissues are harvested, typically under sterile conditions, although the FDA does not require this.[3] The procurement and testing process typically requires about 14 days in full.

After the procurement process, the donor tissue must be stored for use. There are differing opinions as to the optimal temperature and medium to store allografts. In the past, some tissue banks used to deep freeze their grafts up to temperatures greater than $-40°C$.[3] It is now known that fresh OCA material, as opposed to frozen tissue, provides improved viability of chondrocytes. Furthermore, recent laboratory studies suggest that storage at body temperature ($37°C$) enhances chondrocyte viability compared with storage at $4°C$.[9,10] The counterargument to storing at higher temperatures puts grafts at risk for spoilage as well as infection as bacteria grow faster at warmer temperatures.[11] Most tissue banks store the graft tissue at $4°C$. Qi and colleagues[11] showed improved chondrocyte viability in OCAs when the storage medium was refreshed every 2 days as compared with grafts stored in a medium that was not refreshed.

Grafts are typically available for implantation up to the 28-day post harvest time. Effectively, this gives a 2-week window between the completion of procurement and testing up to the 28-day mark. Storing OCAs at $4°C$ slows the metabolism of chondrocytes, which allows for the grafts prolonged shelf life.[9] This system, however, has accumulative detrimental effects on chondrocyte viability, especially in the superficial zone of cartilage. Studies have shown that after 28 days at $4°C$, the chondrocytes have lost enough viability that the graft incorporation is affected.[12,13] Despite these recent reports, others have shown successful clinical and radiographic outcomes in OCAs transplanted after the recommended 28-day mark.[14,15]

Previous biochemical studies have shown that several proapoptotic genes are upregulated in stored OCAs, including tumor necrosis factor-alpha.[16] Linn and colleagues[17] proposed that storage of OCAs in a medium with etanercept, a potent tumor necrosis factor-alpha inhibitor, may prolong chondrocyte viability during storage. The results of their controlled laboratory experiment were promising, showing significantly higher levels of viable chondrocytes in goat allografts stored in the etanercept medium. This finding may be able to prolong shelf life of OCAs, providing a longer window of time to match grafts for recipients.[18]

TECHNICAL CONSIDERATIONS

When considering the use of an OCA, the surgeon must consider the indications listed previously. Once a patient is determined to be a candidate, an OCA may be requested from the tissue bank. Typically, the allografts come specific for the site of injury, that is, for a medial femoral condyle lesion, the graft would be a distal femur graft. As mentioned, there is 2-week window that a graft is available; therefore, the patient and surgeon must be available on short notice.

The surgeon must thoroughly evaluate the cartilage defect typically with arthroscopy; whether this is done before requesting an OCA is surgeon preference. Many surgeons perform a first look, or typically these patients have undergone previous procedures that document the cartilage defect. Inspection can be carried out with the standard arthroscopy. Once visualized, the defect should be measured for size and depth. At this point, it is determined whether to carry out implantation by arthroscopy or if the lesion would better be addressed by arthrotomy.

There are 2 basic types of implantation, the shell and the dowel technique. The original method of implantation is the shell technique, where the graft and recipient site were prepared free hand. With advancements in technology, the dowel technique was designed, which uses cylindrical tools to allow precision press-fitting of these OCAs. The dowel technique does require that the graft be inserted perpendicular to the articular surface, which may require a more extensive exposure.

Although the shell technique requires recipient site preparation with a series of curettes, the dowel technique uses a K-wire and series of reamers to get down to healthy bleeding bone, typically 6 to 12 mm (**Fig. 2**).[18]

Once the recipient site is prepped and measured, attention is turned to the OCA. Articular congruence must be taken into consideration, because recession is better tolerated than elevation of a graft (**Fig. 3**). Nakagawa and colleagues[19] showed that up to 1 mm of graft recession had acceptable outcomes. Alternatively, grafts left elevated even only 1 mm showed increased contact pressures of more than 20% of normal. This can lead to long-term degenerative changes of the joint.[20,21]

Meticulous surgical technique is essential in OCA harvesting and implantation. Previous studies have shown that aggressive drilling or overuse of the mallet can result in cellular damage or necrosis to chondrocytes.[22,23] Recent improvement in instrumentation allows the surgeon to press-fit the graft with greater precision to minimize impaction, which can create impulses great enough to lead to chondrocyte apoptosis.[24]

OUTCOMES

Despite improvements in graft procurement, storage, and surgical technique, OCA transplantation is still mainly used as a salvage procedure. Higher failure rates have

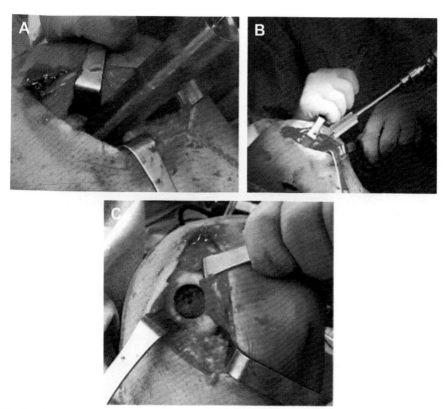

Fig. 2. The dowel technique of a lateral femoral condyle lesion. The K-wire is inserted into the center of the lesion. Reamers were used to create a circular area of healthy bleeding bone and vertical walls. This makes for the ideal recipient site. (*A*) Guide to measure and center the K-wire is inserted. (*B*) Once the pin is placed, reamers are used to create a circular recipient site. (*C*) The final recipient site after reaming.

been related to chronic steroid use, treatment of larger more complex lesions, revision procedures, bipolar or kissing lesions, overweight or obese patients, limb malalignment, inflammatory arthropathies, immunocompromised patients, advancing age, and patients with concomitant ligamentous injury, meniscal insufficiency, or patellofemoral disease.[25]

Documented failure rates vary in the current literature and are heavily dependent on anatomic location. Additionally, there is no standard measure of failure, making reporting outcomes difficult. The lowest failure rates have been documented in femoral condyle transplants with reports ranging from 0% to 22%.[13,26] Saltzman and associates reported[27] failure rates as high as 50% in humeral head transplants. Various other reports of failure rates at other sites include the talar dome (28%),[28] bipolar tibiotalar implants (29%),[29] knee transplants with associated meniscal transplant (22.9%),[30] and distal metatarsal transplant (0%).[31] Most of these are small case series that do not have a standardized measure of failure versus success nor a verified timeframe to consider treatment a failure.

Evaluating survivorship is an alternative way to determine outcomes, although these studies were also limited by patient size and ill-defined parameters for success versus failure (**Table 1**).

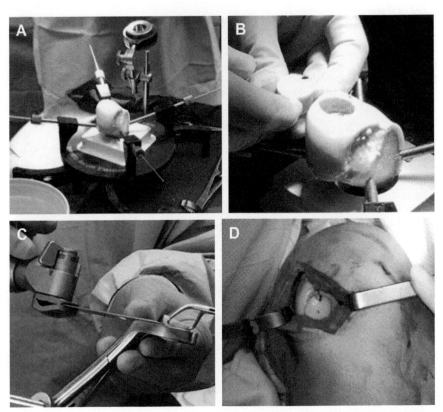

Fig. 3. Preparation and insertion of the osteochondral allograft. (*A*) A device that allows positioning of the donor graft to allow proper harvesting of a graft appropriately sized and contoured to the recipient site. (*B*) The osteochondral allograft has been prepared to match the recipient site. (*C*) The final depth of the graft can be adjusted to ensure that it will not sit proud in the joint. (*D*) The osteochondral allograft has been inserted into the appropriate position, ensuring that it does not sit proud.

Table 1
Survivorship of osteochondral allografts

Site	5-y Survivorship (%)	10-y Survivorship (%)	15-y Survivorship (%)
Tibiotalar joint[29]	76	44	NA
Knee after subchondral marrow stimulation[32]	NA	82	74.9
Knee combined with meniscal transplant[30]	73	68	NA
Revision of the knee[33]	79	61	NA
Distal femoral[26,a]	—	91	84
Isolated patella[32]	78.1	78.1	55.8

[a] This study also included 69% and 59% at 20 and 25 years, respectively.

In the study by Gracitelli and colleagues,[32] which was a level 4 case series of 28 knees with isolated patellar defects, despite having reoperation rates of more than 60%, pain and function improved overall and nearly 90% of patients reported they were satisfied with their outcomes. The reported allograft survivorship in this study was 78.1% at 5 years and 55.8% at 15 years. This suggests that OCAs can provide an acceptable option for salvage treatment, even in patellar chondral defects.

Surface cartilage restoration techniques, such as autologous chondrocyte implantation, have higher reoperation rates for clinical and radiographic graft failures, especially after subchondral marrow stimulation procedures. Thus, the advantages of OCAs seem to correlate with the ability to reconstitute the entire cartilage–subchondral bone unit. OCAs avoid cystic formation, osseous overgrowth, and development of a tougher subchondral plate, all of which can be detrimental to the cartilage–subchondral bone unit.[32]

As with other outcome measures, functional outcomes of OCAs are difficult to interpret owing to the wide variety of scales used. Additionally, subjective scales of patient-reported satisfaction may be biased and not entirely revealing. Regardless of the difficulties in ascertaining patient outcomes, it is apparent that patients whose grafts that were considered successful radiographically generally report that they are satisfied with their outcomes and show improvement on most functional scales.[26]

A recent comparative analysis by Ding and colleagues[34] looked at the biochemical properties of OCAs as compared with diseased articular cartilage. The grafts demonstrated significantly lower levels of proteoglycan-depleting metalloproteinases. This outcome suggests that the composition of the OCAs have a better potential to preserve their tissue quality. These findings also imply that limiting inflammation in the joint may help to improve the outcome and survival of the graft.

When transplanting any tissue, there is typically an inflammatory reaction. This can be related to the donor-recipient blood type or HLA compatibility. Currently, donors and recipients are not matched with regard to these components. This lack of matching can lead to prolonged inflammatory responses and have deleterious effects on the graft incorporation and survivorship. Although not everyone will produce antibodies against the HLAs, studies have shown that as many as 70% of patients who received large allografts and 54% of patients who received medium sized allografts produced these antibodies. Patients who produce higher amounts of antibodies have been shown to have worse clinical outcomes.[22]

Despite the promising results of these studies, many of these patient will go on to develop some degree of long-term arthritis. Even with incorporation of OCAs, potential complications include subsidence, resorption, and in some cases, necrosis.[35] Once again, it seems that the best use of OCAs is as a salvage procedure, which is generally performed to delay arthroplasty or arthrodesis of a joint.

It is important to realize that OCA procedures can make subsequent surgeries more difficult and potentially less successful. Morag and colleagues[36] reported a retrospective review of 35 knees in patients who underwent total knee arthroplasty with a history of previous OCA. At the time of arthroplasty, they found more technical challenges such as patients requiring a more extensive exposure, a greater degree of constraint of prosthesis, and increased need for bone graft. They also found a greater rate of earlier revision as compared with standard total knee arthroplasties.

Cryopreserved Viable Osteochondral Allograft: Shell Allograft

Newer products have been created in an effort to surpass the limitations of fresh allografts, such as their 28-day shelf life, their rigid contour, and difficulty inserting with an arthroscopic approach. Cryopreserved viable osteochondral allografts (CVOCAs) are designed with pores to limit the quantity of bone and enhance their flexibility. This allows the grafts to adapt to different contours on the articular surface. The pores also allow improved penetration of the preservative used to store the grafts allowing them to be frozen for up to 2 years.[37,38] CVOCAs are typically used in combination with marrow stimulation techniques, such as microfracture, which allows mesenchymal stem cells to penetrate the pores in the graft leading to chondrogenesis and production of type II collagen. Although the data are limited regarding CVOCAs, a study by Geraghty and colleagues[38] shows promising outcomes from this technique.

SURGICAL CONSIDERATIONS

Geraghty and colleagues[38] describe their process for making the CVOCAs. Grafts were taken from healthy cartilage of donor knees. Plugs ranged from 1 to 3 mm thick and were 10 and 20 mm in diameter. The majority of the bone was removed from the grafts, leaving full-thickness articular cartilage and subchondral bone. Pore sizes varied using 0.6 and 0.9 mm diameters and densities of 12, 25, and 50 pores/cm^2. They found the best flexibility of the grafts with 0.9 mm diameter pores with density of 50 pores/cm^2. They ultimately chose grafts with 1-mm diameter pores with a density of 36 pores/cm^2.

OUTCOMES

Further in vitro testing of CVOCAs with pores produced more chondrogenic growth factor transforming growth factor-β1 than those without pores, likely owing to the increase in surface area.[38] CVOCAs also produced several transforming growth factors and bone morphogenic proteins at a statistically higher rate than flash frozen OCAs.[39] Most important, in vivo testing of goat models demonstrated the ability for CVOCAs to reestablish type II collagen within the repair site.[38]

FUTURE DIRECTIONS

The use of CVOCAs is relatively new and more research is required. Although preliminary in vitro testing and animal studies show promising results, more data are needed for human outcomes with regard to indications, maximum defect size, rehabilitation, and outcomes.

Particulated Articular Cartilage: Paste Autograft/Allograft

One of the more recent advances in cartilage preservation is in the form of transplanting particulated articular cartilage into a defect that has the ability to create hyaline-like cartilage, which can integrate into the surrounding host tissue. Although autologous chondrocyte implantation techniques require 2-staged procedures, these techniques offer a single-staged implantation of allograft tissue and can account for some of the shortcomings of OCAs (ie, incorporation of implanted bone, the technical challenge of matching the allograft in size and curvature to the host defect). These new methods were based on the assumption that chondrocytes could be implanted and incorporated without an underlying bony support. This has been born out in studies, which have found that, when cartilage is minced into small fragments (1-2 mm^2), chondrocytes within the area were able to migrate out of their initial extracellular matrix and begin to multiply and form a new hyaline-like tissue that integrated into surrounding tissues.[40] Additionally, the scaffolds stimulate the adult stem cells to differentiate into chondrogenic cells. The initial studies in the United States investigated the implantation of transplanted autograft cartilage (Cartilage Autograft Implantation System [CAIS; DePuy/Mitek, Raynham, MA]). This was followed up by similar studies using juvenile cartilage allograft, which had the advantage of decreasing complications associated with harvest. Additionally, it is felt that juvenile cartilage has a greater propensity for cellular activity than aged cartilage. The tissue is harvested from donors 13 years of age or younger because this age groups has been shown to have higher levels of type II collagen and proteoglycan production.[41] Animal models yielded positive results leading to the FDA classifying DeNovo NT (Zimmer, Warsaw, IN) in the same class as osteochondral and other tendon allografts. Similarly, dehydrated cartilage scaffolds such as BioCartilage (Arthrex Inc., Naples, FL) have been shown to stimulate stem cells toward a chondrogenic pathway. Each of these techniques allows for a single-staged procedure to address chondral defects as opposed to procedures that require culturing of autologous chondrocytes with subsequent implantation at a later procedure (eg, Carticel [Genzyme Corp., Cambridge, MA]).[42] Recently, cartilage in vitro bioengineering studies have investigated which characteristics are more likely to promote chondrogenesis, finding that a combination of small scaffold pores with overall low porosity yields lower oxygen tension and allows appropriate transport of nutrients to promote chondrogenesis.[43]

INDICATIONS

Indications for these procedures are controversial and not, at this point, agreed upon across the board. Some suggest that relative indications include International Cartilage Repair Society grade III or higher lesion from 1 to 5 cm in size in a ligamentously stable knee with an intact meniscus and no malalignment. Relative contraindications include bipolar lesions, significant subchondral edema, or an OCD lesion with more than 6 mm of subchondral bone loss.

TECHNICAL CONSIDERATIONS

Initial autograft techniques (ie, CAIS) required harvest of hyaline cartilage from low load-bearing surfaces; these newer techniques have the benefit of avoiding taking intact cartilage from the patient. After a diagnostic arthroscopy, a small arthrotomy can be performed, if necessary, to visualize the lesion directly. The lesion is then outlined with a scalpel or sharp curette along with burrs or shavers to create a shoulder of intact cartilage perpendicular to the surface of the bone. Curettes are then used to remove any remaining cartilage down through the calcified zone in the area of the defect. Although some investigators maintain that the subchondral bone should not be violated, others recommend microfracture if bleeding is not visualized in the defect.[44] A piece of sterile aluminum foil can be pressed into the prepared defect to create a mold, which is then measured. One package of DeNovo covers 2.5 cm^2. The particulated cartilage is distributed onto the mold and a fibrin glue is then added and allowed to cure, after turning off the irrigation (if performing arthroscopically) and drying the defect, the patch is then place into the defect with additional glue added to the surface of the bone.[40] Others have suggested that the graft can be placed directly into the defect followed by the application of the fibrin glue.[45] Some promote mixing the graft with platelet-rich plasma before coating with the fibrin glue,[44] although no studies have investigated whether any of these techniques is superior.

REHABILITATION

There is no consensus on postoperative rehabilitation. However, it is widely accepted that chondrocytes thrive in an environment with adequate compressive and shear forces, which promote protein translation. In vitro studies have shown that dynamic, simulated compression and shear forces provoke cellular outgrowth and long-term chondrogenic maturation at the messenger RNA level compared with samples that did not undergo simulated compression and shear forces. However, type II collagen was weaker in the cultures that underwent simulated compression and shear forces. An increasing number of similar studies hope to provide insight into the delicate balance of maintaining chondrocyte health while avoiding excessive forces that compromise graft incorporation and growth.[46]

Most protocols involve placing the patient into a hinged knee brace after the procedure and using continuous passive motion out of the brace early in the recovery (usually after 1 week). The early stages (weeks 1–6) emphasize protection of the graft to allow the scaffold to stabilize. Protocols differ based on the location of the lesion, with trochlear lesions generally allowing safe immediate weight bearing as tolerated in extension and condylar or plateau lesions requiring a period of non–weight bearing initially (usually 2 weeks). Humeral or glenoid lesions generally require 1 to 2 weeks of complete immobilization followed by progression to range of motion only for 6 weeks.[42] Generally, low load activities are resumed at between 6 weeks and 3 months with gradual progression.[47]

OUTCOMES

Biocartilage in addition to microfracture has been shown to be superior than microfracture alone in animal studies in terms of integration with surrounding cartilage, integration with bone, and collagen type II synthesis.[44] Long-term follow-up studies are limited, but so far have had promising results.

Most reports are single patient or small cohorts but have shown resolution of subchondral bone edema, MRI with fill of defect, and significant improvement in pain and function on clinical scales at up to 2 years of follow-up.[48] Thirteen patients with patellar lesions treated at the University of Iowa had improvements in Knee Injury and Osteoarthritis Outcome Score pain subscales, activities of daily living, and subjective symptoms at an average of 8.2 months' follow-up.[49] An ongoing, multicenter, prospective, single arm study of 25 subjects has reported outcomes on 4 patients who have completed 12 months of follow-up revealing Knee Injury and Osteoarthritis Outcome Score, IKDS and visual analogue scale scores had all improved at 12 months.[50] Case reports have also suggested that the procedure can be effective for talar defects with improvement in pain and function at 2 years postoperatively.[45]

In terms of histologic analysis, a recent report detailed the case of a 44-year-old woman who initially underwent a high tibial osteotomy with de novo repair of a medial femoral condyle lesion after 2 meniscectomies. She had persistent pain with workup revealing an adjacent chondral defect with subsequent OATS procedure performed adjacent to the initial lesion. She ultimately underwent unicondylar knee arthroplasty at 28 months after her initial procedure, allowing microscopic analysis of the integrated particulated graft. Although the patient ultimately required additional procedures, the ability to evaluate the graft material in a human subject revealed that the new cartilage incorporated well with dense proteoglycan content and seemed to be hyaline-like under polarized light.[41]

Ultimately, although clinical outcomes have been promising, long-term comparative studies are needed to help develop indications and postoperative protocols, and to compare these techniques with other available joint preservation techniques.

INFECTION

One major concerns of allograft use, as highlighted by the previously mentioned American Orthopaedic Society for Sports Medicine survey, is the risk of disease transmission. Although numerous studies have investigated the incidence of bacterial infection after transplantation of allograft tissue, there are challenges associated with differentiating standard postoperative infections from ones directly associated from bacteria within the graft. In the 1980s, Tomford and colleagues[51] documented a 6.9% incidence of infection from allografts. Over the years, improved storage, screening, and handling techniques have lowered the reported infection rate. The complexity of the situation is that contamination can occur during handling of an otherwise sterile allograft. In contrast, recognizing viral transmission has been somewhat easier, although reporting of these incidences has been variable in the past. In either case, there is no validated reporting system for infections related to allografts.

BACTERIAL TRANSMISSION

Staphylococcus infection is the most common bacteria responsible for donor tissue contamination.[52] Additionally, *Clostridium* species, commonly found among intestinal flora, are another bacterium recognized in allograft infections. There is a general consensus that between 24 and 48 hours after death bacteria from the intestinal flora transmigrate into the surrounding tissue, blood, and potential donor sites. Therefore, it is common practice to harvest the donor tissue within 24 hours of death.[6] A report from the Centers for Disease Control and Prevention in 2002 reported 26 total bacterial cases from allografts, 13 of which were attributed to *Clostridium*. The same report also identified that 11 cases were a combination of gram-negative bacilli, polymicrobial flora, or culture negative.[53] Malinin and colleagues[6] reviewed nearly 800 cadaveric donors and found that contamination can be detected in blood, bone marrow, as well as the potentially donated tissue. Therefore, they concluded that multiple cultures should be done routinely for all donors.

VIRAL TRANSMISSION

Donor screening with blood testing and questionnaires as well as NAT have proved to effectively to eliminate high-risk donors and significantly decreased the rate of transmission. Since 2005, when the AATB implemented NAT for HIV and HCV, there have been no reported cases of transmission of these viruses.[7]

The first reported case of HIV transmission from allograft tissue was in 1988 and the last reported case of HIV transmission from allograft tissue occurred in 1996 with an untested donor.[54]

HCV transmission in the past was commonly owing to donors initially testing negative. Tugwell and coworkers[55] reported a case in which a donor tested negative for antibodies against HCV and this tissue was used for donation. After 8 patients subsequently were infected with HCV, the donor was later found to be positive for HCV RNA. This led to a more rigorous testing protocol for HCV to include HCV RNA.[55]

The first reported transmission of human T-cell lymphotropic virus was in 1991. The recipient patient remained asymptomatic despite showing antibodies against human T-cell lymphotropic virus.[56]

There is no specific protocol for testing for Zika virus in regard to allograft use. In early 2016, the FDA released recommendations with regard to screening and deferral of potential donors specific to blood transfusions. They recommend that all potential donors be screened for Zika virus using questionnaires regarding travel and symptoms as well as obtaining whole blood tests. Any symptomatic donor is deferred for at least 4 weeks after the resolution of symptoms. Although we are still continuing to try to understand the Zika virus, orthopedists must be cognizant of the potential harms from this unfamiliar and evolving situation.[57]

SUMMARY

With the continuously increasing life expectancy, there is a growing demand for joint preservation techniques to delay joint replacements, especially in the younger active patients. Ideally, techniques would recreate the natural articular hyaline cartilage of the joint while allowing the patient to return to their preinjury functional level. This article highlights the nature of articular injuries as well as several options for treatment. Options like microfracture show acceptable outcomes for smaller lesions up to 2 cm^2, although this technique results in healing of the defect with fibrocartilage, a less advantageous alternative. Autologous chondrocyte implantation shows promising results for cartilage defects up to 4 cm^2, although it requires a minimum of 2 procedures. OCAs provide a viable option for larger defects, joints with multiple defects, or joints that have failed other cartilage procedures. With improving and continually evolving techniques of storage and focus on preserving the viability of chondrocytes, allografts have shown encouraging outcomes. Newer techniques like CVOCAs and particulated grafts allow for longer shelf life and flexibility to adapt to various defects of articular cartilage. The majority of the papers presented show low failure rates, improving survivorship, and promising functional outcomes. Future direction of research will need to focus on prolonging shelf life of allografts, enhancing incorporation of grafts, and improving viability of chondrocytes at the time of implantation.

REFERENCES

1. Lexer E. Substitute of whole or half-joints from freshly amputated extremities by free plastic operation. Surg Gynecol 1908;6:601–7.
2. AOSSM. 2006 AOSSM orthopaedic surgical procedure survey on allografts. Naperville (IL): Leever Research Services; 2006.
3. McAllister DR, Joyce MJ, Mann BJ, et al. Allograft update: the current status of tissue regulation, procurement, processing, and sterilization. Am J Sports Med 2007;35(12):2148–58.
4. Gudas R, Kalesinskas RJ, Kimtys V, et al. A prospective randomized clinical study of mosaic osteochondral autologous transplantation versus microfracture for the treatment of osteochondral defects in the knee joint in young athletes. Arthroscopy 2005;21(9):1066–75.
5. Food and Drug Administration (FDA). Guidance for Industry Current Good Tissue Practice (CGTP) and additional requirements for manufacturers of human cells, tissues, and cellular and tissue-based products (HCT/Ps). vol. 4. Rockville (MD): Food and Drug Administration; 2009.
6. Malinin TI, Buck BE, Temple HT, et al. Incidence of clostridial contamination in donors' musculoskeletal tissue. J Bone Joint Surg Br 2003;85(7):1051–4. Available at: http://www.ncbi.nlm.nih.gov/pubmed/14516045. Accessed July 30, 2016.
7. Vaishnav S, Vangsness T, Dellamaggiora R. New techniques in allograft tissue processing. Clin Sports Med 2009;28(1):127–41.
8. Veen MR, Bloem RM, Petit PL. Sensitivity and negative predictive value of swab cultures in musculoskeletal allograft procurement. Clin Orthop Relat Res 1994; 300:259–63. Available at: http://www.ncbi.nlm.nih.gov/pubmed/8131346. Accessed July 30, 2016.
9. Pallante AL, Bae WC, Chen AC, et al. Chondrocyte viability is higher after prolonged storage at 37 degrees C than at 4 degrees C for osteochondral grafts. Am J Sports Med 2009;37(Suppl 1):24S–32S.

10. Bastian JD, Egli RJ, Ganz R, et al. Chondrocytes within osteochondral grafts are more resistant than osteoblasts to tissue culture at 37°C. J Invest Surg 2011; 24(1):28–34.

11. Qi J, Hu Z, Song H, et al. Cartilage storage at 4 °C with regular culture medium replacement benefits chondrocyte viability of osteochondral grafts in vitro. Cell Tissue Bank 2016;17(3):473–9.

12. Ball ST, Amiel D, Williams SK, et al. The effects of storage on fresh human osteochondral allografts. Clin Orthop Relat Res 2004;418:246–52. Available at: http://www.ncbi.nlm.nih.gov/pubmed/15043126. Accessed July 30, 2016.

13. LaPrade RF, Botker J, Herzog M, et al. Refrigerated osteoarticular allografts to treat articular cartilage defects of the femoral condyles. A prospective outcomes study. J Bone Joint Surg Am 2009;91(4):805–11.

14. Drobnic M, Radosavljevic D, Cör A, et al. Debridement of cartilage lesions before autologous chondrocyte implantation by open or transarthroscopic techniques: a comparative study using post-mortem materials. J Bone Joint Surg Br 2010;92(4): 602–8.

15. Mithoefer K, Williams RJ, Warren RF, et al. The microfracture technique for the treatment of articular cartilage lesions in the knee. A prospective cohort study. J Bone Joint Surg Am 2005;87(9):1911–20.

16. Robertson CM, Allen RT, Pennock AT, et al. Upregulation of apoptotic and matrix-related gene expression during fresh osteochondral allograft storage. Clin Orthop Relat Res 2006;442:260–6. Available at: http://www.ncbi.nlm.nih.gov/pubmed/16394770. Accessed July 30, 2016.

17. Linn MS, Chase DC, Healey RM, et al. Etanercept enhances preservation of osteochondral allograft viability. Am J Sports Med 2011;39(7):1494–9.

18. Torrie AM, Kesler WW, Elkin J, et al. Osteochondral allograft. Curr Rev Musculoskelet Med 2015;8(4):413–22.

19. Nakagawa Y, Suzuki T, Kuroki H, et al. The effect of surface incongruity of grafted plugs in osteochondral grafting: a report of five cases. Knee Surg Sports Traumatol Arthrosc 2007;15(5):591–6.

20. Harris JD, Solak KK, Siston RA, et al. Contact pressure comparison of proud osteochondral autograft plugs versus proud synthetic plugs. Orthopedics 2011; 34(2):97.

21. Johnson MR, LaPrade RF. Tibial plateu "Kissing Lesion" from a proud osteochondral autograft. Am J Orthop (Belle Mead NJ) 2011;40(7):359–61. Available at: http://www.ncbi.nlm.nih.gov/pubmed/22013573. Accessed July 30, 2016.

22. Bugbee WD, Pallante-Kichura AL, Görtz S, et al. Osteochondral allograft transplantation in cartilage repair: graft storage paradigm, translational models, and clinical applications. J Orthop Res 2016;34(1):31–8.

23. Bisicchia S, Rosso F, Amendola A. Osteochondral allograft of the talus. Iowa Orthop J 2014;34:30–7. Available at: http://www.ncbi.nlm.nih.gov/pubmed/25328456. Accessed July 30, 2016.

24. Giannini S, Buda R, Pagliazzi G, et al. Survivorship of bipolar fresh total osteochondral ankle allograft. Foot Ankle Int 2014;35(3):243–51.

25. Khanna V, Tushinski DM, Drexler M, et al. Cartilage restoration of the hip using fresh osteochondral allograft: resurfacing the potholes. Bone Joint J 2014; 96-B(11 Supple A):11–6.

26. Raz G, Safir OA, Backstein DJ, et al. Distal femoral fresh osteochondral allografts: follow-up at a mean of twenty-two years. J Bone Joint Surg Am 2014;96(13): 1101–7.

27. Saltzman B, Riboh J, Cole B, et al. Humeral head reconstruction with osteochondral allograft transplantation. Arthroscopy 2015;31(9):1827–34.

28. Haene R, Qamirani E, Story RA, et al. Intermediate outcomes of fresh talar osteochondral allografts for treatment of large osteochondral lesions of the talus. J Bone Joint Surg Am 2012;94(12):1105–10.

29. Bugbee WD, Khanna G, Cavallo M, et al. Bipolar fresh osteochondral allografting of the tibiotalar joint. J Bone Joint Surg Am 2013;95(5):426–32.

30. Getgood A, Gelber J, Gortz S, et al. Combined osteochondral allograft and meniscal allograft transplantation: a survivorship analysis. Knee Surg Sports Traumatol Arthrosc 2015;23(4):946–53.

31. Ajis A, Seybold JD, Myerson MS. Osteochondral distal metatarsal allograft reconstruction: a case series and surgical technique. Foot Ankle Int 2013;34(8):1158–67.

32. Gracitelli GC, Meric G, Briggs DT, et al. Fresh osteochondral allografts in the knee: comparison of primary transplantation versus transplantation after failure of previous subchondral marrow stimulation. Am J Sports Med 2015;43(4):885–91.

33. Horton MT, Pulido PA, McCauley JC, et al. Revision osteochondral allograft transplantations: do they work? Am J Sports Med 2013;41(11):2507–11.

34. Ding L, Zampogna B, Vasta S, et al. Why do osteochondral allografts survive? comparative analysis of cartilage biochemical properties unveils a molecular basis for durability. Am J Sports Med 2015;43(10):2459–68.

35. Shasha N, Aubin PP, Cheah HK, et al. Long-term clinical experience with fresh osteochondral allografts for articular knee defects in high demand patients. Cell Tissue Bank 2002;3(3):175–82.

36. Morag G, Kulidjian A, Zalzal P, et al. Total knee replacement in previous recipients of fresh osteochondral allograft transplants. J Bone Joint Surg Am 2006;88(3):541–6.

37. Ohlendorf C, Tomford WW, Mankin HJ. Chondrocyte survival in cryopreserved osteochondral articular cartilage. J Orthop Res 1996;14(3):413–6.

38. Geraghty S, Kuang J-Q, Yoo D, et al. A novel, cryopreserved, viable osteochondral allograft designed to augment marrow stimulation for articular cartilage repair. J Orthop Surg Res 2015;10(1):66.

39. Fortier LA, Barker JU, Strauss EJ, et al. The role of growth factors in cartilage repair. Clin Orthop Relat Res 2011;469(10):2706–15.

40. Farr J, Cole BJ, Sherman S, et al. Particulated articular cartilage: CAIS and DeNovo NT. J Knee Surg 2012;25(1):23–9. Available at: http://www.ncbi.nlm.nih.gov/pubmed/22624244. Accessed November 25, 2016.

41. Stevens HY, Shockley BE, Willett NJ, et al. Particulated juvenile articular cartilage implantation in the knee: a 3-year EPIC- CT and histological examination. Cartilage 2014;5(2):74–7.

42. Hirahara AM, Mueller KW. BioCartilage: a new biomaterial to treat chondral lesions. Sports Med Arthrosc 2015;23(3):143–8.

43. Nava MM, Draghi L, Giordano C, et al. The effect of scaffold pore size in cartilage tissue engineering. J Appl Biomater Funct Mater 2016;14(3):e223–9.

44. Fortier LA, Chapman HS, Pownder SL, et al. BioCartilage improved cartilage repair compared with microfracture alone in an equine model of full-thickness cartilage loss. Am J Sports Med 2016;44(9):2366–74.

45. Kruse DL, Ng A, Paden M, et al. Arthroscopic De Novo NT® juvenile allograft cartilage implantation in the talus: a case presentation. J Foot Ankle Surg 2012;51(2):218–21.

46. Wang N, Grad S, Stoddart MJ, et al. Particulate cartilage under bioreactor-induced compression and shear. Int Orthop 2014;38(5):1105–11.
47. Cole BJ, Farr J, Winalski CS, et al. Outcomes After a Single-Stage Procedure for Cell-Based Cartilage Repair: a prospective clinical safety trial with 2-year follow-up. Am J Sports Med 2011;39(6):1170–9.
48. Bonner KF, Daner W, Yao JQ. 2-year postoperative evaluation of a patient with a symptomatic full-thickness patellar cartilage defect repaired with particulated juvenile cartilage tissue. J Knee Surg 2010;23(2):109–14. Available at: http://www.ncbi.nlm.nih.gov/pubmed/21141688. Accessed November 25, 2016.
49. Buckwalter JA, Bowman GN, Albright JP, et al. Clinical outcomes of patellar chondral lesions treated with juvenile particulated cartilage allografts. Iowa Orthop J 2014;34:44–9. Available at: http://www.ncbi.nlm.nih.gov/pubmed/25328458. Accessed November 25, 2016.
50. Farr J, Yao JQ. Chondral defect repair with particulated juvenile cartilage allograft. Cartilage 2011;2(4):346–53.
51. Tomford WW, Starkweather RJ, Goldman MH. A study of the clinical incidence of infection in the use of banked allograft bone. J Bone Joint Surg Am 1981;63(2):244–8. Available at: http://www.ncbi.nlm.nih.gov/pubmed/7007391. Accessed July 30, 2016.
52. Stepanović ŽL, Ristić BM. Bacterial infections associated with allogenic bone transplantation. Vojnosanit Pregl 2015;72(5):427–30. Available at: http://www.ncbi.nlm.nih.gov/pubmed/26165050. Accessed July 30, 2016.
53. Centers for Disease Control and Prevention (CDC). Update: allograft-associated bacterial infections–United States, 2002. MMWR Morb Mortal Wkly Rep 2002;51(10):207–10. Available at: http://www.ncbi.nlm.nih.gov/pubmed/11922189. Accessed July 31, 2016.
54. Hinsenkamp M, Muylle L, Eastlund T, et al. Adverse reactions and events related to musculoskeletal allografts: reviewed by the World Health Organisation Project NOTIFY. Int Orthop 2012;36(3):633–41.
55. Tugwell BD, Patel PR, Williams IT, et al. Transmission of hepatitis C virus to several organ and tissue recipients from an antibody-negative donor. Ann Intern Med 2005;143(9):648–54. Available at: http://www.ncbi.nlm.nih.gov/pubmed/16263887. Accessed July 31, 2016.
56. Sanzén L, Carlsson A. Transmission of human T-cell lymphotrophic virus type 1 by a deep-frozen bone allograft. Acta Orthop Scand 1997;68(1):72–4. Available at: http://www.ncbi.nlm.nih.gov/pubmed/9057574. Accessed July 31, 2016.
57. Food and Drug Administration (FDA). Recommendations for donor screening, deferral, and product management to reduce the risk of transfusion- transmission of Zika virus guidance for industry. Rockville (MD): US Dep Heal Hum Serv Food Drug Adm Cent Biol Eval Res; 2016.

Autologous Chondrocytes and Next-Generation Matrix-Based Autologous Chondrocyte Implantation

 CrossMark

Betina B. Hinckel, MD, PhD[a], Andreas H. Gomoll, MD[b],*

KEYWORDS

- Knee • Cartilage • Cartilage repair • Autologous chondrocyte implantation
- Transplantation • Autologous • Chondrocytes/*transplantation • Articular/*surgery

KEY POINTS

- Identify type of lesion (traumatic or idiopathic).
- Evaluate associated lesions (malalignment, meniscal lesion, and ligamentous instability).
- Long length alignment radiograph and MRI are important complementary studies.
- Conservative measures should be exhausted before proceeding with surgical treatment.
- Autologous chondrocyte implantation is indicated for the treatment of medium to large, full-thickness cartilage defects (>2 cm^2).

INTRODUCTION

Focal chondral defects of the knee are common and can significantly impair quality of life. Studies have demonstrated chondral or osteochondral lesions in up to 61% to 66% of patients undergoing knee arthroscopy.[1–3] A recent systematic review estimated the overall prevalence of focal chondral defects of the knee specifically in athletes to be 36%.[4] However, the true incidence and prevalence is difficult to determine because a large percentage of defects are asymptomatic. If left untreated, these defects can lead to osteoarthritis.[5,6]

Surgical techniques to restore articular cartilage have the goal to increase quality of life by improving pain and function, and also potentially delay or prevent the need for knee arthroplasty. Autologous chondrocyte implantation (ACI) was first described in 1994.[7] It is a 2-stage procedure: the first procedure includes the arthroscopic

[a] Missouri Orthopaedic Institute, University of Missouri, Virginia Avenue, Columbia, MO, USA;
[b] Cartilage Repair Center, Brigham and Women's Hospital, Chestnut Hill, MA, USA
* Corresponding author.
E-mail address: AGOMOLL@BWH.HARVARD.EDU

Clin Sports Med 36 (2017) 525–548
http://dx.doi.org/10.1016/j.csm.2017.02.008
0278-5919/17/© 2017 Elsevier Inc. All rights reserved.

evaluation of the chondral defect(s) and an articular cartilage biopsy, and the second stage is the implantation of the cultured chondrocytes.

The ACI technique has evolved over the past 20 years: the first-generation technique involved the use of a periosteal patch (pACI) harvested from the proximal tibia.[7] This early periosteal patch technique resulted in a high rate of graft hypertrophy often requiring reoperation for arthroscopic debridement.[8,9] The second-generation technique (cACI) uses a type I/III collagen membrane The newest third-generation technique seeds and cultivates the collagen membrane with chondrocytes before implantation and is referred to as matrix-induced autologous chondrocyte implantation (MACI).[10] These techniques and their outcomes are discussed in this article.

PATIENT EVALUATION OVERVIEW
Clinical Evaluation: History and Physical Examination

Unfortunately, neither history nor clinical examination is sensitive or specific for cartilage defects versus other intra-articular derangements, such as meniscal tears.

Clinical complaints:

- Knee pain: important to identify location (medial, lateral, anterior, or posterior), position of the knee (flexion or extension), and situations that increase or decrease pain (weight-bearing vs non–weight-bearing, stairs vs flat ground, specific activities).
- Swelling: important to know degree, frequency, and related activities.
- Mechanical symptoms: catching and locking may be present as well as a feeling of instability.

Traumatic etiologies are often associated with a specific event, such as a fall or twisting injury during sports; for example, patellar dislocation, ACL tear, or direct blunt force trauma. Idiopathic lesions and those associated with repetitive microtrauma may have more of an insidious onset without an event the patient can recall.

Physical examination:

- Gait analysis
- Tibiofemoral malalignment and patellar maltracking (static varus or valgus, dynamic valgus with single leg squat; increased Q-angle and rotational malalignment, with increased femoral anteversion and in-toe or out-toe pattern)
- Patellar malalignment/maltracking (lateral position and lateral tilt, patella alta; and J-sign and subluxation with quadriceps contraction in extension)
- Muscle strength, flexibility, and atrophy (core: abdomen, dorsal and hip muscles; and lower limb: quadriceps, hamstrings, and gastrocnemius)
- Effusion
- Crepitus
- Active and passive range of motion (spine, hips, and both knees)
- Location of pain/tenderness to palpation (medial, lateral, distal, or retropatellar)
- Ligamentous and soft tissue stability/imbalance (tibiofemoral and patellar: apprehension, glide test, and tilt test)

Imaging

Imaging studies allow characterization of the lesions, identification of associated lesions (ligaments and meniscus), and alignment. In the tibiofemoral joint, the alignment is evaluated by the mechanical axis. Tibial or femoral deformities should be noted. Patellofemoral joint alignment is evaluated by patellar height, tilt, and tibial-tubercle trochlear-groove distance (TT-TG).

- Routine knee radiograph (anteroposterior, lateral, merchant, and 45-degree flexion posteroanterior weight-bearing views): evaluate for fractures, loose bodies, osteophytes, and joint space narrowing.
- Full limb length radiographs: determine mechanical axis alignment.
- Computed tomography (CT): provide fine anatomic detail of subchondral bone when bone injury is suspected; for example, after subchondral drilling, bone grafting, or osteochondral allograft transplantation, as well as for osteochondritis dissecans (OCD) or osteochondral fracture. The addition of intra-articular contrast (CT arthrogram) allows for excellent visualization of the articular cartilage.
- MRI: evaluate articular cartilage, soft tissues, and bone marrow lesions (subchondral edema). Estimate the grade and the size of the lesion to guide treatment, although MRI frequently underestimates lesion size by up to 60%.[11]

Treatment

The initial management for most articular cartilage lesions consists of rest, activity modification, anti-inflammatory medications, and physical therapy. Generally, conservative measures should be exhausted (between 3 and 6 months) before proceeding with surgical treatment. The threshold for indicating surgery is lower in traumatic lesions in young patients and higher in older patients with idiopathic lesions.

Nonsurgical Treatment Options

Injections in the form of corticosteroids or viscosupplementation may help decrease inflammation and improve symptoms in certain patients, especially older individuals with degenerative disease with the goal of bridging to arthroplasty.

An unloader brace can be effective in cases of unilateral compartment overload in which a chondral defect is exposed to excessive forces as a result of malalignment or meniscal deficiency. For the patellofemoral joint, bracing or taping can be used to unload the affected site.

SURGICAL TREATMENT
Indications

ACI is indicated for the treatment of medium to large, full-thickness cartilage defects. Due to the cost and invasiveness of the procedure, ACI is a second-line treatment for defects smaller than 2 cm,[12] in which it is generally reserved for revision of prior failed cartilage repair. For larger defects, however, it can be used as a primary procedure due to the lowered efficacy of lesser procedures, such as microfracture or osteochondral autograft transfer.

The extensive postoperative recovery and rehabilitation after ACI, delayed return to sports and heavy labor, as well as permanent restrictions/recommendations require a careful preoperative discussion with the patient and family to establish reasonable expectations and avoid disappointment.

Contraindications include active or recent infection, inflammatory arthritis, significant medical comorbidities, and inability to follow the complex postoperative rehabilitation. Uncontained and bipolar lesions are a relative contraindication and require special techniques. Articular comorbidities are a common cause of chondral defects, and potential failure mechanism after cartilage repair. As such, lower extremity malalignment, ligamentous instability, patellofemoral instability and maltracking, stiffness, and meniscal insufficiency are not absolute contraindications to ACI, but require careful preoperative assessment and treatment in a staged or concomitant fashion.

SURGICAL PROCEDURE
Arthroscopic Assessment and Biopsy

The knee joint is examined under anesthesia to assess ligamentous stability, range of motion, crepitation, and patellar mobility and tracking.

Arthroscopy is performed to assess the overall condition of the knee joint, as well as to specifically evaluate the menisci for current tears or prior resection. The articular surfaces are then evaluated for any defect(s). It is important to note the size and location of the defects as well as plan how to access the lesion using an open approach for the implantation procedure. Quality and thickness of the surrounding and opposing cartilage should be carefully assessed specifically for uncontained and bipolar defects.

If the arthroscopic assessment is favorable for ACI treatment, a cartilage biopsy is obtained. The cartilage is usually harvested from the superior and lateral aspect of the intercondylar notch. In case of a prior anterior cruciate ligament reconstruction notchplasty, this area is frequently overgrown with fibrocartilage, which should *not* be harvested (medial aspect of the notch or periphery of the trochlea should be harvested instead). A gouge or curette is used to mobilize a strip of cartilage 5 mm wide and 10 to 15 mm long (200–300 mg). It is left attached at one end to avoid losing the biopsy in the joint (**Fig. 1**). It is then removed with the tissue grasper or pituitary rongeur and directly placed in sterile transport medium for shipment.

Chondrocytes Culture

The biopsy is placed in cryopreservation where it can remain for up to 5 years. Once the implant procedure has been scheduled, the cells are removed from cryopreservation, thawed, and cultured for an additional 3 to 4 weeks. A standard order can yield up to 4 vials of 12 million cells each, contained in 0.4 mL of culture media. Additional vials can be special ordered for multiple and large defects, but require additional cell passage, adding additional cost and time. Generally, the recommendation is to use 1 vial

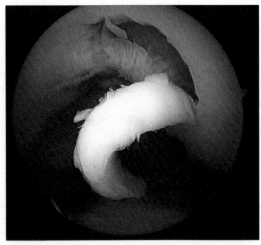

Fig. 1. Cartilage biopsy. Arthroscopic view of cartilage biopsy of the superior and lateral portion of intercondylar notch. (*Courtesy of* Andreas Gomoll, MD, Brigham and Women's Hospital, Chestnut Hill, MA.)

of cells per defect and to aim for a seeding density of 1 to 2 million cells per square centimeters. The cells are delivered the day before or day of the procedure and expire within 48 hours.

Implantation Technique

Except for patch preparation, fixation, and chondrocyte implantation, the procedure is identical for ACI and MACI.

Exposure

Adequate exposure is critical to ensure appropriate defect preparation and implant placement.

- Femoral condyle: Isolated lesions are accessible through a limited medial or lateral arthrotomy without violating the extensor mechanism. Multiple and larger lesions require more extensile approaches, including larger parapatellar or subvastus approaches. Correct placement of retractors is crucial, especially in limited incisions. We routinely place a bent Hohmann retractor into the notch, displacing the patella, while a Z-retractor is placed peripherally around the condyle to retract the capsule. Posterior lesions may require an approach similar to the one for the tibia.
- Patella: Requires patellar eversion, through either a parapatellar incision into the quadriceps tendon, or a subvastus approach for mobilization of the extensor mechanism.
- Tibia: May require mobilization of the anterior meniscal horn, either by transection of the anterior root or osteotomy of a small bone block at the root insertion, with subsequent repair at the end of the procedure.

Defect preparation

Careful defect preparation is critical and all degenerated cartilage should be removed to achieve a stable rim with vertical shoulders (**Fig. 2**). The defect is outlined with a fresh scalpel down to the subchondral plate, taking as much of the surrounding cartilage to remove all unstable or undermined cartilage. The degenerated cartilage is debrided with small ring or conventional curettes; however, if this would transform a peripheral defect from a contained to an uncontained lesion, it is advisable to leave a small rim of degenerated cartilage to sew into. The debridement includes the zone of calcified cartilage, but maintains an intact subchondral plate. Minor punctate bleeding is frequently encountered but can usually be controlled with fibrin glue or epinephrine-soaked neuropatties. The tourniquet should be released during defect preparation to visualize and address any potential bleeding.

Patch preparation, fixation, and chondrocyte implantation

Autologous chondrocyte implantation The lesion is templated with a sterile marking pen and tracing paper. Our preference is to cut the collagen membrane dry according to the template (**Fig. 3**), and then the porous side is seeded with the chondrocyte solution. Generally, the dry patch will readily absorb the cell suspension, and after a 5-minute period to allow the cells to preliminarily attach to the membrane, the patch can be placed into the defect. It is placed on the defect with the porous side toward the bone. The patch is sutured tight enough to not sit on the bone but rather be flush with the surrounding cartilage, creating a space underneath to inject the chondrocyte suspension. Resorbable 6 to 0 suture on a cutting needle, immersed in mineral oil or glycerin for handling, is used for suturing. The sutures are placed through the patch and then the articular cartilage, exiting approximately 3 mm away from the defect edge, everting

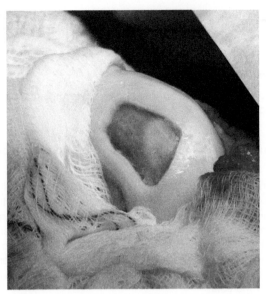

Fig. 2. Debrided cartilage defect. Cartilage should be removed to achieve a stable rim with vertical shoulders. (*Courtesy of* Andreas Gomoll, MD, Brigham and Women's Hospital, Chestnut Hill, MA.)

the edge of the patch slightly to provide a better seal against the defect wall. The knots are tied on the patch side, seated below the level of the adjacent cartilage (**Fig. 4**). The suture line is waterproofed with fibrin glue. An opening wide enough to accept an angiocath is left in the most superior aspect of the patch to inject the chondrocytes (see **Fig. 4**); this opening is closed with additional suture and fibrin glue after the defect has been completely filled with chondrocyte suspension.

Matrix-induced autologous chondrocyte implantation For MACI, the chondrocytes are delivered on a preseeded collagen membrane (**Fig. 5**). The membrane is sized according to the template, then placed with the porous side facing the subchondral bone. The edges are trimmed to ensure there is no prominence that could

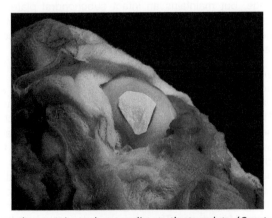

Fig. 3. Collagen membrane. It is cut dry according to the template. (*Courtesy of* Andreas Gomoll, MD, Brigham and Women's Hospital, Chestnut Hill, MA.)

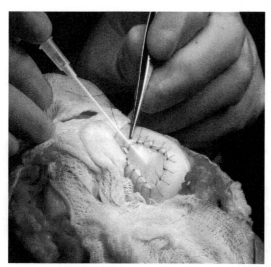

Fig. 4. Fixation of the membrane and chondrocyte injection. The knots are tied on the patch side, seated below the level of the adjacent cartilage and chondrocytes are injected through an opening in the most superior aspect of the patch that is subsequently closed with additional suture and fibrin glue. (*Courtesy of* Andreas Gomoll, MD, Brigham and Women's Hospital, Chestnut Hill, MA.)

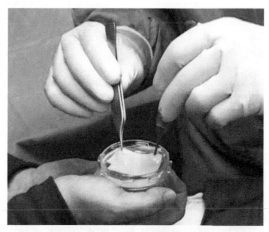

Fig. 5. Matrix-induced autologous chondrocyte implantation membrane. (*Courtesy of* Seth L. Sherman, MD, University of Missouri, Columbia, MO.)

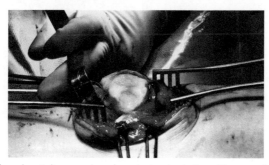

Fig. 6. Matrix-induced autologous chondrocyte implantation. The membrane is implanted in medial and lateral patellar facets defects, fixed by fibrin glue. (*Courtesy of* Seth L. Sherman, MD, University of Missouri, Columbia, MO.)

compromise the mechanical stability of the implant during range of motion. The membrane is then secured with either fibrin glue only (**Fig. 6**), or additional sutures can be placed around the periphery if there are concerns for stability. The knee is then ranged to ensure secure fixation.

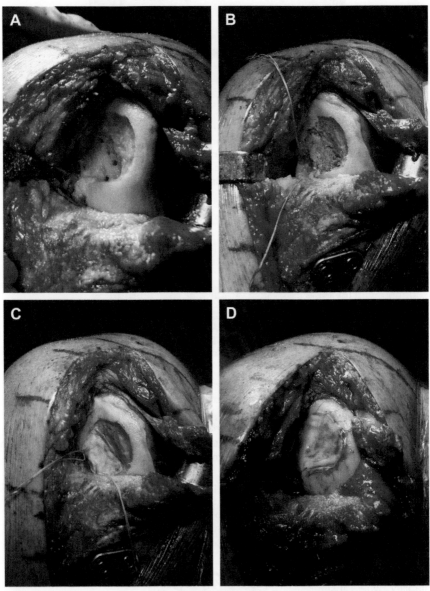

Fig. 7. Grafting of osteochondral lesion with "sandwich" technique. (*A*) Debrided osteochondral defect, a deeper osseous defect can be appreciated at the inferolateral aspect of the defect. (*B*) Bone loss has been grafted up to the subchondral level. (*C*) Membrane is covering the bone grafting. (*D*) Final appearance with sutured membrane over the cartilage defect. (*Courtesy of* Andreas Gomoll, MD, Brigham and Women's Hospital, Chestnut Hill, MA.)

For ACI or MACI we minimize the use of intra-articular drains to avoid damage to the patch. When drains are used, it should be without suction and with care to position the tubing away from the defect.

Special Situations

Osteochondral lesions: Bony defects deeper than 6 to 8 mm should be considered for staged or concomitant autologous bone grafting (**Fig. 7**) from the proximal tibia or distal femur.

Uncontained defect: Membrane should be fixed by transosseous sutures or small suture anchors to ensure mechanical stability.

Intralesional osteophytes (**Fig. 8**): Should be burred down to the level of the surrounding subchondral plate with a high-speed bur under constant cold irrigation.

Rehabilitation

Immediate motion is encouraged. A continuous passive motion machine is used 6 to 8 hours a day for the first 6 weeks. The motion is progressed toward 90° over the first 2 to 3 weeks. The patient remains toe-touch weight bearing for a minimum of 6 weeks. At 7 weeks, the patient starts to progress toward weight bearing as tolerated. Running is restricted for 12 months and most strenuous cutting activities for 18 months until the graft has fully matured.

TREATMENT RESISTANCE/COMPLICATIONS

Standard complications of knee surgery include deep vein thrombosis, wound infection, arthrofibrosis, and neurovascular injury. Complications specific to ACI include failure to form an appropriate repair tissue (biologic failure) and delamination of a well-formed graft (mostly traumatic failure).

EVALUATION OF OUTCOME AND LONG-TERM RECOMMENDATIONS

Clinical evidence is extensive and includes long-term follow-ups (over 10 years) of case series[13–17] and randomized controlled trials (RCTs),[18,19] and also many systematic reviews and meta-analyses.[20–26]

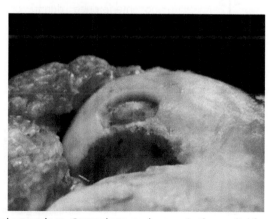

Fig. 8. Intralesional osteophyte. Osteophyte can be seen in the medial femoral condyle after initial debridement of the lesion. (*Courtesy of* Andreas Gomoll, MD, Brigham and Women's Hospital, Chestnut Hill, MA.)

Table 1
Clinical studies: autologous chondrocyte implantation (ACI) and matrix-induced autologous chondrocyte implantation (MACI)

Procedure	Author (Year)	Study Type (Number of Subjects)	Age	Defect Location/Size	Follow-Up	Results and Comments
pACI and OAT	Horas et al,[36] 2003	RCT pACI (20) vs OAT (20)	Mean 31.4 y	Knee, all locations/ 3.75 cm^2	2 y	Both treatments resulted in a decrease in symptoms. ACI improvement lagged behind OAT. Histology: ACI with fibrocartilage and OAT retained hyaline cartilage with a persistent interface between the transplant and the surrounding original cartilage. More women in ACI group and more men in OAT group.
pACI/cACI and OAT	Bentley et al,[37] 2003	RCT pACI (58) vs OAT (42)	Mean 31.3 y	Knee, all locations/ mean 4.66 cm^2	Mean 19 mo	Modified Cincinnati and Stanmore scores and objective clinical assessment showed that 88% had excellent or good results after ACI compared with 69% after OAT. Arthroscopy (at 1 y) excellent or good repairs in 82% after ACI and in 34% after OAT.
pACI and MFx	Knutsen et al,[28] 2004	RCT pACI (40) vs MFx (40)	Mean 33.3 y (ACI) and 31.1 y (MFx)	Knee, femoral condyles/mean 5.1 cm^2 (ACI) and 4.5 cm^2 (MFx)	2 y	Small differences between 2 groups with both groups having significant clinical improvement. With MFx, smaller lesions (<4 cm^2) had better clinical results. No difference with ACI. With both treatments, younger patients (<30 y) had better clinical outcomes. Histology: no significant differences between the 2 groups.

pACI	Minas and Bryant,[41] 2005	Case series (45)	Mean 37.5 y	Knee, patellofemoral/patella 4.86 cm² and trochlea 5.22 cm²	>2 y, mean 46 mo	71% patients rated outcome good or excellent, 22% as fair, and 7% as poor. Knee Society Score improved from 53 to 74, Modified Cincinnati improved from 3.84 to 5.76.
cACI and MACI	Bartlett et al,[12] 2005	RCT cACI (44) vs MACI (47)	Mean 33.7 y in cACI and 33.4 y in MACI	Knee, all locations/mean 6 cm² in cACI and 6.1 cm² in MACI	1 y	Clinical improvement in both groups. Modified Cincinnati improved by 17.6 in the cACI and 19.6 in MACI. Arthroscopy: ICRS good to excellent in 79.2% of cACI and 66.6% of MACI. Histology: Hyalinelike cartilage or hyalinelike cartilage with fibrocartilage in 43.9% of cACI and 36.4% of MACI. Hypertrophy of the graft was 9% in cACI group and 6% in MACI. Reoperation was 9% in each group.
cACI	Micheli et al,[42] 2006	Case series (37): children and adolescents	Mean 16 y	Knee, femoral condyles/mean 5.4 cm²	>2 y, mean 4.3 y	Knee score improved from 3.4 ± 1.6 to 7.2 ± 2.4. Knee pain improved from 3.1 ± 2.5 to 7.1 ± 3.0.
ACI	Knutsen et al,[27] 2007	RCT ACI (40) vs MFx (40)	No data	Knee, femoral condyle/no data on size	5 y	Satisfactory results in 77%. No difference in the Lysholm or VAS pain between groups. One-third of patients with early radiographic signs of osteoarthritis (no difference between groups). Failures: 9 (23%) in each group.
pACI	Mandelbaum et al,[43] 2007	Case series (40): 48% after failed MFx	Mean 37.1 y	Knee, trochlea/mean 4.5 cm²	Mean 59 ± 18 mo	13% associated Fulkerson procedure. Modified Cincinnati improved from 3.1 ± 1.0 to 6.4 ± 1.7. 11 patients experienced 17 subsequent procedures (adhesions in 4 cases, periosteal flap detachment in 4 cases, chondromalacia in 4 cases).

(continued on next page)

Table 1
(continued)

Procedure	Author (Year)	Study Type (Number of Subjects)	Age	Defect Location/Size	Follow-Up	Results and Comments
pACI and cACI	Niemeyer et al,[45] 2008	Case series (70)	Mean 34.3 y	Knee, patella/mean 4.41 ± 2.15 cm²	Mean 38.4 mo	Lysholm 73.0 ± 22.4 and IKDC 62 ± 21.5 at follow-up (no preoperative data). Better results at lateral facet lesions. Cincinnati sports activity improvement from 34.4 ± 33.9 to 61.5 ± 21.5.
pACI	Rosenberger et al,[46] 2008	Case series (56): >45 y	Mean 48.6 y	Knee, all locations/means 4.7 cm² per defect and 9.8 cm² per knee	Mean 4.7 y	Failures: 8 failures total 14%. Additional arthroscopy: 24 patients (43%) for periosteal-related problems and adhesions; 88% of these patients experienced lasting improvement. 81% of patients would again undergo ACI.
pACI and MACI	Ferruzzi et al,[47] 2008	Comparative study open pACI (48) vs arthroscopic MACI (50)	Mean 31.5 y	Knee, femoral condyles/mean 6.4 cm² (ACI) and 5.9 cm² (MACI)	>5 y	IKDC improvement in both treatments with no significant differences between them. More rapid improvement with arthroscopic MACI. Tissue regeneration, remodeling, and integration with the adjacent tissue in 89% (ACI) and 93% (MACI).
pACI	Minas et al,[44] 2009	Case series (325):	Mean 35 y	Knee, all locations/mean 8.2 cm²	Mean 55 mo	111 previous MFx and 214 no previous MFx. Failures: 26% with previous MFx and 8% without previous MFx (3 times more failures in MFx).
cACI	Saris et al,[35] 2009	RCT ACI (57) vs MFx (61)	Mean 33.9 y	Knee, single femoral condyle/mean 2.5 cm²	3 y	Greater KOOS improvement in ACI (21.25 ± 3.60) than in MFx (15.83 ± 3.48). Subchondral bone reaction significantly worsened over time with MFx compared with ACI.

cACI	Zaslav et al,[9] 2009	Case series (124): all with failed previous cartilage procedure (debridement and MFx)	Mean 34.5 y	Knee, all locations/ mean 4.63 ± 3.20 cm²	4 y	67% treatment successes and 24% failures. 49% had subsequent surgical procedures. Modified Cincinnati improvement from 3.3 to 6.3. Similar results for previous MFx and debridement.
MACI	Gobbi et al,[48] 2009	Case series (34)	Mean 31.2 y	Knee, patellofemoral/ mean 4.45 cm²	>5 y	Significant improvement at 2 and 5 y. IKDC improvement from 46.09 ± 19.3 to 77.06 ± 17.0 at 2 y and 70.39 ± 21.4 at 5 y. Biopsy samples with hyaline-line.
MACI and Mfx	Kon et al,[33] 2009	RCT ACI (40) vs MFx (40)	Mean 29.8 y	Knee, femoral condyles or trochlea/2.4 cm²	>5 y	MACI significantly more effective than MFx. IKDC improvement: MACI from 40.5 ± 15.2 to 80.2 ± 19.1 and MFx 41.1 ± 12.3 to 70.2 ± 14.7.
pACI	McNickle et al,[49] 2009	Case series (140)	Mean 30.3 y	Knee, all locations/ mean 5.2 ± 3.5 cm²	Mean 4.3 y	75% patients were completely or mostly satisfied; 83% would have the procedure again. IKDC improvement from 34 to 64, and Lysholm improvement from 41 to 69. 16% required ACI debridement postoperatively. Failures: 6.4%. Age and workers' compensation are independent predictors of outcomes.
pACI	Moseley et al,[14] 2010	Case series (72)	Mean 37 y	Knee, all locations/ mean 5.2 ± 4.15 cm²	>10 y	Survivorship: 83%. 87% improved from 5 y to 10 y; 69% improved from baseline to 10 y. Failures 17% (75% of failures occurred at average 2.5 y). Operations after ACI: 42%.

(continued on next page)

Table 1
(continued)

Procedure	Author (Year)	Study Type (Number of Subjects)	Age	Defect Location/Size	Follow-Up	Results and Comments
pACI	Peterson et al,[16] 2010	Case series (224)	Mean 33.3 y	Knee, all locations/ mean 5.3 cm²	10–20 y, mean 12.8 y	74% status as better or the same and 92% would do surgery again. Lysholm improvement: from 60.3 to 69.5. Tegner improvement: from 7.2 to 8.2. Bipolar lesions had worse final outcomes than multiple unipolar lesions. Meniscal injuries, previous marrow procedures, and age did not affect final outcomes.
pACI and MACI	Zeifang et al,[50] 2010	RCT pACI (10) vs MACI (11)	Mean 29.3 y	Knee, all locations/ mean 4.1 ± 09 cm²	2 y	No difference in IKDC, Tegner, and SF-36. pACI better on Lysholm and Gillquist score. Intact subchondral bone seen earlier and more frequently in MACI, and granulations, tissue cysts, or sclerosis seen more frequent in the pACI. 5 women on MACI and none on pACI.
MACI	Niemeyer et al,[51] 2010	Case series (59)	Mean 37.02 y	Knee, all locations/ mean 4.64 cm²	2 y	Patients with ICRS clinical normal and nearly normal increased from 33.9% to 92.5% ACT-CS IKDC 50.1 ± 13.4 to 76.1 ± 15.2 and Lysholm from 60.5 ± 9.4 to 82.5 ± 13.7. Failure: highest at 2 y (26.7%) in salvage procedures, and 5.9% in isolated defects.
MFx and cACI	Van Assche et al,[30] 2010	RCT ACI (33) vs MFx (34)	Mean 31 y	Knee, femoral condyles/mean 2.4 ± 1.5 cm²	2 y	70% of all patients returned to > 85% symmetry in functional performance. ACI resulted in slower recovery. Similar functional outcomes between ACI and MFx.

	Author	Study type (n)	Age	Location/size	Follow-up	Results
MFx and MACI	Basad et al,[31] 2010	RXT MACI (33) vs MFx (15)	Between 18 and 50 y	Knee, all locations/ MACI 2 x the size MFx group	2 y	MACI significantly more effective than MFx. Lysholm improvement: MACI from 52 to 92 and MFx 55 to 69.
cACI and MACI	Macmull et al,[52] 2011	Case series (31)	Mean 16.3 y	Knee, all locations	Mean 66.3 mo	Modified Cincinnati improvement from 48 to 92. VAS pain improvement from 5.0 to 1.5.
cACI and MACI	Kon et al,[53] 2011	Case series (61)	>40 y, mean 45 y	Knee, femoral condyles/mean 2.9 ± 1.2 cm^2	Mean 5 y	IKDC improvement from 36.8 ± 8.4 to 68.1 ± 21.8. Failures: 20%.
MACI	Ebert et al,[54] 2011	Case series (46)	Between 10 and 69 y	Knee, all locations/ from 1 cm^2 to >5 cm^2	5 y	Improvement in all Knee injury and Osteoarthritis Outcome Score and SF-36 subscales as well as the 6-min walk test and active knee extension. MRI: good to excellent fill graft was 77%, 84%, 86%, and 67% (3 mo, 12 mo, 24 mo, and 5 y, respectively). Signal intensity was good to excellent in 23%, 72%, 94%, and 96% (3 mo, 12 mo, 24 mo, and 5 y, respectively). No correlations existed between clinical and MRI-based outcome measures.
pACI	Cole et al,[67] 2012	Case series (40): at least 1 failed non-ACI for OCD	Mean 30.5 y	Knee, femoral condyles and trochlea/mean 5.4 cm^2 per lesion, mean 1.4 lesions per knee; mean 6.3 cm^2 total	Mean 48 mo	85% ACI treatment success. Modified Cincinnati improved from 3.1 ± 1.1 to 6.8 ± 2.0; SF-36 improved from 35.4 to 45.5. Failure: 19%.
pACI, OAT and MFx	Lim et al,[29] 2012	Comparative study pACI (18), OAT (22), and MFx (30)	Mean pACI (25.1 y), OAT (30.4 y), and MFx (32.9 y)	Knee, femoral condyles/mean pACI (2.84 cm^2), OAT (2.75 cm^2),	>3 y, mean 5 y	All procedures improved in functional outcome. No differences between groups. Lysholm: pACI (from 52.4 ± 6.4 to 84.6 ± 6.1), OAT (from 53.2 ± 7.2 to 84.8 ± 5.5), and MFx (51.2 ± 6.2 to 85.6 ± 6.8).

(continued on next page)

Table 1
(continued)

Procedure	Author (Year)	Study Type (Number of Subjects)	Age	Defect Location/Size	Follow-Up	Results and Comments
				and MFx (2.77 cm²)		ICRS Grades 1 or 2: MFx (80%), OAT (82%), and pACI (80%).
cACI	Vanlauwe et al,[55] 2012	Case series (38 total; patella 28, trochlea 7, and both 3)	Mean 30.9 y	Knee, patellofemoral/ 4.89 cm²	>2 y, mean 37 mo	15 patients had a previous or concomitant procedure because of malalignment. VAS pain improvement from 62.1 to 27.4. KOOS improvement from 73.6 ± 19.1. Failures: 5. Adverse events: joint crepitation (18) and arthrofibrosis (7).
MACI	Marlovits et al,[56] 2012	Case series (21)	Mean 35.2 y	Knee, all locations/ mean 5.1 cm²	5 y	KOOS improved from 29.6 ± 9.15 to 77.7 ± 21.2. IKDC improved from 30.1 ± 6.6 to 74.3 ± 20.4. MOCART improved from 52.9 to 75.8 ± 18.0 MRI: complete filling (83%) and integration (82%). Signs of subchondral bone edema were still present in 47%
cACI and OAT	Bentley et al,[18] 2012	RCT cACI (58) vs OAT (42)	Mean cACI (30.9 y) and OAT (31.6 y)	Knee all locations/ mean cACI (4.40 cm²) and OAT (3.99 cm²)	Between 10 and 12 y	cACI better outcomes Cincinnati from nonfailed: cACI (excellent/ good: 73%). OAT (excellent/good: 60%). Failures: cACI (17%) and OAT (55%).
NeoCart (MACI) and MFx	Crawford et al,[32] 2012	RCT NeoCart (21) vs MFx (9)	Mean NeoCart 41 y and MFx 39 y	Knee, femoral condyles/mean NeoCart (2.87 ± 1.38 cm²) and MFx (2.52 ± 1.35 cm²)	2 y	Both groups improved with better improvement on NeoCart for SF-36 and IKDC. More NeoCart were therapeutic responders at 6 mo (43% vs 25% MFx) and 12 mo (76% vs 22% MFx).

	Study	Case series	Mean age	Location/lesion	Follow-up	Outcomes
pACI and BMSC	Teo et al,[57] 2013	Case series (23 total; 20 ACI and 3 BMSC) - OCD	Mean 16.8 y	Knee, patella/no data	Mean 72 mo	Mean IKDC score, Tegner-Lysholm outcomes, and Lysholm-Gillquist scale improved from 45, 2.5, and 50, respectively, to 75, 4, and 70.
pACI	Gomoll et al,[58] 2014	Case series (110)	Mean 33 y	Knee, patella/mean 5.4 ± 2.7 cm²	Mean 90 mo	IKDC improved from 40 ± 14 to 69 ± 20. Cincinnati improvement from 3.2 ± 1.2 to 6.2 ± 1.8. Failures: 8%.
pACI	Minas et al,[13] 2014	Case series (210)	Mean 36 y	Knee, all locations/ mean 8.4 ± 5.5 cm² (1.7 lesions per knee)	>10 y, mean 12 y	Survivorship: 79% at 5 y, and 71% at 10 y. Improved function: 75% (WOMAC 39 ± 21 to 23 ± 16, Knee Society Score from 54 ± 18 to 79 ± 19). Failures: 25%. Increased failure risk with previous MFx and lesion >15 cm².
pACI and cACI	Nawaz et al,[59] 2014	Case series (827)	Mean 34 y	Knee, all locations/ mean 4.09 cm²	Mean 6.2 y	Survivorship: 78% at 5 y and 51% beyond 10 y. VAS pain improvement: from 5.95 to 3.56. Modified Cincinnati improvement: from 46.91 to 66.74. Lateral femoral condyle procedures survived the longest. 5 times failure rate with previous procedure (excluding debridement), such as MFx. No increase in failures with larger lesions.
pACI	Niemeyer et al,[15] 2014	Case series (70)	Mean 33.3 y	Knee, all locations/ mean 6.5 ± 4.0 cm²	Mean 10.9 y	VAS pain improvement from 7.2 ± 1.9 to 2.1 ± 2.1. Lysholm improvement from 42.0 ± 22.5 to 71.0 ± 17.4.

(continued on next page)

Table 1
(continued)

Procedure	Author (Year)	Study Type (Number of Subjects)	Age	Defect Location/Size	Follow-Up	Results and Comments
MACI	Edwards et al,[60] 2014	Comparative study arthroscopic (41) vs open (37)	Mean 35.5 y	Knee, femoral condyles/mean 2.73 cm^2 arthroscopic and 3.02 cm^2 open	From 3 mo to 12 mo	Arthroscopic reduced length of patient hospitalization, and reduced risk of postsurgery complications. No significant difference on MRI.
MACI	Filardo et al,[61] 2014	Case series (133)	No data	Knee all locations/ 2.3 ± 1.0 cm^2	From 1 y to 7 y	IKDC improved from 39.6 ± 14.4 to 71.9 ± 19.8 at 1 y; a further improvement was observed at 2 y (77.0 ± 20.5) and stable over time up to 7 y (77.4 ± 22.1).
MACI	Saris et al,[34] 2014	RCT MACI (72) vs MFx (72)	Mean 33.8 y	Knee, all locations/ mean 4.8 cm^2	2 y	MACI with better outcomes. Modified Cincinnati improved from 3.0 ± 1.2 to 6.4 ± 2.1 on MACI and from 3.0 ± 1.2 to 5.4 ± 2.2 on MFx. IKDC from 32.9 ± 13.3 to 65.7 ± 18.5 on MACI and from 29.3 ± 13.4 to 58.8 ± 22.3 on MFx.
MACI	Basad et al,[66] 2015	Case series (65)	Mean 32 y	No data	From 6 mo to 60 mo	Mean Lysholm score improved from 28.5 to 76.6 points (±19.8) at 24 mo, settling back to 75.5 points after 5 y.
MACI	Ebert et al,[62] 2015	Case series (47 total, 24 patella, 23 trochlea)	Mean 37.5 y	Knee, patellofemoral/ mean 3.3 cm^2	2 y	KOOS improved in all subscales. VAS pain improved from 5.4 ± 1.4 to 1.8 ± 1.1. MRI: 40.4% complete graft infill, 6.4% hypertrophic graft, 31.9% with 50% to 100% graft infill, 17% < 50% tissue infill, and 4.3% graft failure.

	Study	Study Design	Mean Age	Location/Size	Follow-up	Outcomes
cACI	Pestka et al,[64] 2016	Case series (130)	Mean 36.2 y	Knee, all locations/ mean 4.4 ± 1.7 cm²	Mean 5.3 ± 2.3 y	Mean inability to work 13.6 ± 11.0 wk. Return to sports: 73.1%. High-impact as well as start-stop sports were generally substituted for low-intensity exercises.
pACI	Rosa et al,[17] 2016	Case series (15)	Mean 21.3 y	Knee, all location/ mean 5.08 ± 2.01 cm²	Mean 12.3 y	IKDC improvement from 37.20 ± 19.54 to 76.32 ± 32.36 and Tegner from 2.33 ± 1.34 to 4.93 ± 2.43. MRI deterioration: MOCART from 55 ± 26.53 to 45 ± 31.62.
ACI and MFx	Knustsen et al,[19] 2016	RCT ACI (40) vs MFx (40)	No data	Knee, femoral condyle/mean 4.5 cm²	Between 14 and 15 y	Failure: 42.5% in ACI and 32.5% in MFx (difference not significant). 50% of the patients. Nonfailure had early radiographic signs of osteoarthritis, defined as a Kellgren and Lawrence grade of ≥2. Similar in both.
cACI	Cvetanovich et al,[63] 2017	Case series (37)	Mean 16.7 y	Knee, all locations/ mean 4.0 ± 2.2 cm²	Mean 4.6 ± 2.4 y	IKDC subjective improvement from 34.9 to 64.6. Subsequent surgery: 37.8% (most commonly, chondral debridement [54%]).
MACI	Ebert et al,[65] 2017	Case series (31): arthroscopic	Mean 35.3 y	Knee, tibiofemoral/ mean 2.52 cm²	5 y	Lysholm improved from 53.8 ± 6.9 to 86.8 ± 4.2. Tegner improved from 2.7 ± 0.3 to 5.5 ± 0.5. VAS pain improved from 5.7 ± 0.4 to 1.7 ± 0.3. MRI 90% good to excellent tissue infill.

Abbreviations: ACI, autologous chondrocyte implantation; BMSC, bone marrow–derived mesenchymal stem cell; cACI, collagen cover; ICRS, International Cartilage Repair Society; IKDC, International Knee Documentation Committee; KOOS, Knee Injury and Osteoarthritis Outcome Score; MFx, microfracture; MOCART, magnetic resonance observation of cartilage repair tissue; OAT, osteochondral autograft transfer; OCD, osteochondritis dissecans; pACI, periosteum autologous chondrocyte implantation; RCT, randomized controlled trial; SF-36, Short Form-36; VAS, visual analog scale.

RCTs between ACI/MACI and microfracture (MFx) are contradicting. Usually no difference is observed[27–30] when the study is performed for smaller lesions and short follow-ups, whereas better clinical outcomes for ACI/MACI[31–35] are usually associated with larger lesions and longer follow-ups. In RCTs versus OAT (osteochondral autograft transfer) similar results were obtained in some studies,[29,36] with slightly better results for ACI in larger lesions and better results for OAT in smaller lesions.[18,37]

Systematic reviews and meta-analyses are commonly performed for short-term follow-ups, as there are insufficient long-term studies for a meta-analysis. Clinical results are similar among ACI, OAT, and MFx[23,25,26] and better for ACI in one systematic review.[24] Although a systematic review of pediatric patients concluded that MFx, OAT, OCA (osteochondral allograft), and ACI have all been implemented successfully in the pediatric knee, MFx was generally associated with poorer outcomes and shorter durability, particularly in larger lesions (>3 cm^2).[20] In terms of return to sport, the highest rates of returns are after OAT (89% to 93%), followed by OCA (osteochondral allograft) (88%), ACI (82% to 84%), and MFx (58% to 75%).[22,38] Furthermore, hyaline repair tissue was more common with OAT and second-generation ACI than MFx. Even though the clinical significance of this is unknown, this higher-quality tissue may result in increased clinical outcomes and decreased failures rates in the long term.

Data from RCTs and meta-analyses should be considered because most of them are small lesions in the femoral condyles, whereas in clinical setting patients have larger, sometimes multiple lesions and in other locations of the knee.[39]

Among the different generations of ACI (pACI, cACI, and MACI), there is weak evidence that cACI is better than pACI and that MACI is comparable with both.[40] There is good evidence favoring an accelerated weight-bearing regimen after MACI.[40] There is currently no evidence that supports scaffold-based ACI or arthroscopic implantation over first-generation ACI.[40]

Results of most clinically relevant ACI and MACI studies are in **Table 1**.

SUMMARY/DISCUSSION

ACI has been a product approved by the Food and Drug Administration for nearly 20 years with more than 100 publications detailing its efficacy. RCTs have demonstrated improved outcomes against MFx in larger defects, whereas the treatment of small defects generally does not show clinical superiority. It is therefore recommended for the treatment of defects larger than 2 cm[12] in the femoral condyles and trochlea. The patella and tibial plateau are off-label indications, but multiple publications have demonstrated its efficacy, at least for the former, whereas tibial plateau defects are rare. Although cartilage surgery in general, including less-invasive procedures such as marrow stimulation, should include the evaluation and treatment of articular comorbidities such as meniscal deficiency and malalignment, this is of particular importance for more invasive and involved procedures, such as ACI. Newer generations of ACI, such as MACI, allow more minimally invasive approaches, including the potential for arthroscopic defect preparation and graft placement.

REFERENCES

1. Aroen A, Loken S, Heir S, et al. Articular cartilage lesions in 993 consecutive knee arthroscopies. Am J Sports Med 2004;32(1):211–5.
2. Curl WW, Krome J, Gordon ES, et al. Cartilage injuries: a review of 31,516 knee arthroscopies. Arthroscopy 1997;13(4):456–60.
3. Hjelle K, Solheim E, Strand T, et al. Articular cartilage defects in 1,000 knee arthroscopies. Arthroscopy 2002;18(7):730–4.

4. Flanigan DC, Harris JD, Trinh TQ, et al. Prevalence of chondral defects in athletes' knees: a systematic review. Med Sci Sports Exerc 2010;42(10):1795–801.
5. Lefkoe TP, Trafton PG, Ehrlich MG, et al. An experimental model of femoral condylar defect leading to osteoarthrosis. J Orthop Trauma 1993;7(5):458–67.
6. Messner K, Maletius W. The long-term prognosis for severe damage to weight-bearing cartilage in the knee: a 14-year clinical and radiographic follow-up in 28 young athletes. Acta Orthop Scand 1996;67(2):165–8.
7. Brittberg M, Lindahl A, Nilsson A, et al. Treatment of deep cartilage defects in the knee with autologous chondrocyte transplantation. N Engl J Med 1994;331(14): 889–95.
8. Gooding CR, Bartlett W, Bentley G, et al. A prospective, randomised study comparing two techniques of autologous chondrocyte implantation for osteochondral defects in the knee: periosteum covered versus type I/III collagen covered. Knee 2006;13(3):203–10.
9. Zaslav K, Cole B, Brewster R, et al. A prospective study of autologous chondrocyte implantation in patients with failed prior treatment for articular cartilage defect of the knee: results of the Study of the Treatment of Articular Repair (STAR) clinical trial. Am J Sports Med 2009;37(1):42–55.
10. Behrens P, Bitter T, Kurz B, et al. Matrix-associated autologous chondrocyte transplantation/implantation (MACT/MACI)–5-year follow-up. Knee 2006;13(3): 194–202.
11. Gomoll AH, Yoshioka H, Watanabe A, et al. Preoperative measurement of cartilage defects by MRI underestimates lesion size. Cartilage 2011;2(4):389–93.
12. Bartlett W, Skinner JA, Gooding CR, et al. Autologous chondrocyte implantation versus matrix-induced autologous chondrocyte implantation for osteochondral defects of the knee: a prospective, randomised study. J Bone Joint Surg Br 2005;87(5):640–5.
13. Minas T, Von Keudell A, Bryant T, et al. The John Insall award: a minimum 10-year outcome study of autologous chondrocyte implantation. Clin Orthop Relat Res 2014;472(1):41–51.
14. Moseley JB Jr, Anderson AF, Browne JE, et al. Long-term durability of autologous chondrocyte implantation: a multicenter, observational study in US patients. Am J Sports Med 2010;38(2):238–46.
15. Niemeyer P, Porichis S, Steinwachs M, et al. Long-term outcomes after first-generation autologous chondrocyte implantation for cartilage defects of the knee. Am J Sports Med 2014;42(1):150–7.
16. Peterson L, Vasiliadis HS, Brittberg M, et al. Autologous chondrocyte implantation: a long-term follow-up. Am J Sports Med 2010;38(6):1117–24.
17. Rosa D, Balato G, Ciaramella G, et al. Long-term clinical results and MRI changes after autologous chondrocyte implantation in the knee of young and active middle aged patients. J Orthop Trauma 2016;17(1):55–62.
18. Bentley G, Biant LC, Vijayan S, et al. Minimum ten-year results of a prospective randomised study of autologous chondrocyte implantation versus mosaicplasty for symptomatic articular cartilage lesions of the knee. J Bone Joint Surg Br 2012;94(4):504–9.
19. Knutsen G, Drogset JO, Engebretsen L, et al. A randomized multicenter trial comparing autologous chondrocyte implantation with microfracture: long-term follow-up at 14 to 15 years. J Bone Joint Surg Am 2016;98(16):1332–9.
20. Chawla A, Twycross-Lewis R, Maffulli N. Microfracture produces inferior outcomes to other cartilage repair techniques in chondral injuries in the paediatric knee. Br Med Bull 2015;116:93–103.

21. DiBartola AC, Wright BM, Magnussen RA, et al. Clinical outcomes after autologous chondrocyte implantation in adolescents' knees: a systematic review. Arthroscopy 2016;32(9):1905–16.

22. Krych AJ, Pareek A, King AH, et al. Return to sport after the surgical management of articular cartilage lesions in the knee: a meta-analysis. Knee Surg Sports Traumatol Arthrosc 2016. [Epub ahead of print].

23. Mundi R, Bedi A, Chow L, et al. Cartilage restoration of the knee: a systematic review and meta-analysis of level 1 studies. Am J Sports Med 2016;44(7): 1888–95.

24. Oussedik S, Tsitskaris K, Parker D. Treatment of articular cartilage lesions of the knee by microfracture or autologous chondrocyte implantation: a systematic review. Arthroscopy 2015;31(4):732–44.

25. Riboh JC, Cvetanovich GL, Cole BJ, et al. Comparative efficacy of cartilage repair procedures in the knee: a network meta-analysis. Knee Surg Sports Traumatol Arthrosc 2016. [Epub ahead of print].

26. Samsudin EZ, Kamarul T. The comparison between the different generations of autologous chondrocyte implantation with other treatment modalities: a systematic review of clinical trials. Knee Surg Sports Traumatol Arthrosc 2016;24(12): 3912–26.

27. Knutsen G, Drogset JO, Engebretsen L, et al. A randomized trial comparing autologous chondrocyte implantation with microfracture. Findings at five years. J Bone Joint Surg Am 2007;89(10):2105–12.

28. Knutsen G, Engebretsen L, Ludvigsen TC, et al. Autologous chondrocyte implantation compared with microfracture in the knee. A randomized trial. J Bone Joint Surg Am 2004;86-A(3):455–64.

29. Lim HC, Bae JH, Song SH, et al. Current treatments of isolated articular cartilage lesions of the knee achieve similar outcomes. Clin Orthop Relat Res 2012;470(8): 2261–7.

30. Van Assche D, Staes F, Van Caspel D, et al. Autologous chondrocyte implantation versus microfracture for knee cartilage injury: a prospective randomized trial, with 2-year follow-up. Knee Surg Sports Traumatol Arthrosc 2010;18(4):486–95.

31. Basad E, Ishaque B, Bachmann G, et al. Matrix-induced autologous chondrocyte implantation versus microfracture in the treatment of cartilage defects of the knee: a 2-year randomised study. Knee Surg Sports Traumatol Arthrosc 2010; 18(4):519–27.

32. Crawford DC, DeBerardino TM, Williams RJ 3rd. NeoCart, an autologous cartilage tissue implant, compared with microfracture for treatment of distal femoral cartilage lesions: an FDA phase-II prospective, randomized clinical trial after two years. J Bone Joint Surg Am 2012;94(11):979–89.

33. Kon E, Gobbi A, Filardo G, et al. Arthroscopic second-generation autologous chondrocyte implantation compared with microfracture for chondral lesions of the knee: prospective nonrandomized study at 5 years. Am J Sports Med 2009;37(1):33–41.

34. Saris D, Price A, Widuchowski W, et al. Matrix-applied characterized autologous cultured chondrocytes versus microfracture: two-year follow-up of a prospective randomized trial. Am J Sports Med 2014;42(6):1384–94.

35. Saris DB, Vanlauwe J, Victor J, et al. Treatment of symptomatic cartilage defects of the knee: characterized chondrocyte implantation results in better clinical outcome at 36 months in a randomized trial compared to microfracture. Am J Sports Med 2009;37(Suppl 1):10S–9S.

36. Horas U, Pelinkovic D, Herr G, et al. Autologous chondrocyte implantation and osteochondral cylinder transplantation in cartilage repair of the knee joint. A prospective, comparative trial. J Bone Joint Surg Am 2003;85-A(2):185–92.

37. Bentley G, Biant LC, Carrington RW, et al. A prospective, randomised comparison of autologous chondrocyte implantation versus mosaicplasty for osteochondral defects in the knee. J Bone Joint Surg Br 2003;85(2):223–30.

38. Campbell AB, Pineda M, Harris JD, et al. Return to sport after articular cartilage repair in athletes' knees: a systematic review. Arthroscopy 2016;32(4):651–68.e1.

39. Foldager CB, Farr J, Gomoll AH. Patients scheduled for chondrocyte implantation treatment with MACI have larger defects than those enrolled in clinical trials. Cartilage 2016;7(2):140–8.

40. Goyal D, Goyal A, Keyhani S, et al. Evidence-based status of second- and third-generation autologous chondrocyte implantation over first generation: a systematic review of level I and II studies. Arthroscopy 2013;29(11):1872–8.

41. Minas T, Bryant T. The role of autologous chondrocyte implantation in the patellofemoral joint. Clin Orthop Relat Res 2005;(436):30–9.

42. Micheli LJ, Moseley JB, Anderson AF, et al. Articular cartilage defects of the distal femur in children and adolescents: treatment with autologous chondrocyte implantation. J Pediatr Orthop 2006;26(4):455–60.

43. Mandelbaum B, Browne JE, Fu F, et al. Treatment outcomes of autologous chondrocyte implantation for full-thickness articular cartilage defects of the trochlea. Am J Sports Med 2007;35(6):915–21.

44. Minas T, Gomoll AH, Rosenberger R, et al. Increased failure rate of autologous chondrocyte implantation after previous treatment with marrow stimulation techniques. Am J Sports Med 2009;37(5):902–8.

45. Niemeyer P, Steinwachs M, Erggelet C, et al. Autologous chondrocyte implantation for the treatment of retropatellar cartilage defects: clinical results referred to defect localisation. Arch Orthop Trauma Surg 2008;128(11):1223–31.

46. Rosenberger RE, Gomoll AH, Bryant T, et al. Repair of large chondral defects of the knee with autologous chondrocyte implantation in patients 45 years or older. Am J Sports Med 2008;36(12):2336–44.

47. Ferruzzi A, Buda R, Faldini C, et al. Autologous chondrocyte implantation in the knee joint: open compared with arthroscopic technique. Comparison at a minimum follow-up of five years. J Bone Joint Surg Am 2008;90(Suppl 4):90–101.

48. Gobbi A, Kon E, Berruto M, et al. Patellofemoral full-thickness chondral defects treated with second-generation autologous chondrocyte implantation: results at 5 years' follow-up. Am J Sports Med 2009;37(6):1083–92.

49. McNickle AG, L'Heureux DR, Yanke AB, et al. Outcomes of autologous chondrocyte implantation in a diverse patient population. Am J Sports Med 2009;37(7):1344–50.

50. Zeifang F, Oberle D, Nierhoff C, et al. Autologous chondrocyte implantation using the original periosteum-cover technique versus matrix-associated autologous chondrocyte implantation: a randomized clinical trial. Am J Sports Med 2010;38(5):924–33.

51. Niemeyer P, Lenz P, Kreuz PC, et al. Chondrocyte-seeded type I/III collagen membrane for autologous chondrocyte transplantation: prospective 2-year results in patients with cartilage defects of the knee joint. Arthroscopy 2010;26(8):1074–82.

52. Macmull S, Parratt MT, Bentley G, et al. Autologous chondrocyte implantation in the adolescent knee. Am J Sports Med 2011;39(8):1723–30.

53. Kon E, Filardo G, Condello V, et al. Second-generation autologous chondrocyte implantation: results in patients older than 40 years. Am J Sports Med 2011; 39(8):1668–75.

54. Ebert JR, Robertson WB, Woodhouse J, et al. Clinical and magnetic resonance imaging-based outcomes to 5 years after matrix-induced autologous chondrocyte implantation to address articular cartilage defects in the knee. Am J Sports Med 2011;39(4):753–63.

55. Vanlauwe JJ, Claes T, Van Assche D, et al. Characterized chondrocyte implantation in the patellofemoral joint: an up to 4-year follow-up of a prospective cohort of 38 patients. Am J Sports Med 2012;40(8):1799–807.

56. Marlovits S, Aldrian S, Wondrasch B, et al. Clinical and radiological outcomes 5 years after matrix-induced autologous chondrocyte implantation in patients with symptomatic, traumatic chondral defects. Am J Sports Med 2012;40(10): 2273–80.

57. Teo BJ, Buhary K, Tai BC, et al. Cell-based therapy improves function in adolescents and young adults with patellar osteochondritis dissecans. Clin Orthop Relat Res 2013;471(4):1152–8.

58. Gomoll AH, Gillogly SD, Cole BJ, et al. Autologous chondrocyte implantation in the patella: a multicenter experience. Am J Sports Med 2014;42(5): 1074–81.

59. Nawaz SZ, Bentley G, Briggs TW, et al. Autologous chondrocyte implantation in the knee: mid-term to long-term results. J Bone Joint Surg Am 2014;96(10): 824–30.

60. Edwards PK, Ebert JR, Janes GC, et al. Arthroscopic versus open matrix-induced autologous chondrocyte implantation: results and implications for rehabilitation. J Sport Rehabil 2014;23(3):203–15.

61. Filardo G, Kon E, Andriolo L, et al. Clinical profiling in cartilage regeneration: prognostic factors for midterm results of matrix-assisted autologous chondrocyte transplantation. Am J Sports Med 2014;42(4):898–905.

62. Ebert JR, Fallon M, Smith A, et al. Prospective clinical and radiologic evaluation of patellofemoral matrix-induced autologous chondrocyte implantation. Am J Sports Med 2015;43(6):1362–72.

63. Cvetanovich GL, Riboh JC, Tilton AK, et al. Autologous chondrocyte implantation improves knee-specific functional outcomes and health-related quality of life in adolescent patients. Am J Sports Med 2017;45(1):70–6.

64. Pestka JM, Feucht MJ, Porichis S, et al. Return to sports activity and work after autologous chondrocyte implantation of the knee: which factors influence outcomes? Am J Sports Med 2016;44(2):370–7.

65. Ebert JR, Fallon M, Wood DJ, et al. A prospective clinical and radiological evaluation at 5 years after arthroscopic matrix-induced autologous chondrocyte implantation. Am J Sports Med 2017;45(1):59–69.

66. Basad E, Wissing FR, Fehrenbach P, et al. Matrix-induced autologous chondrocyte implantation (MACI) in the knee: clinical outcomes and challenges. Knee Surg Sports Traumatol Arthrosc 2015;23(12):3729–35.

67. Cole BJ, DeBerardino T, Brewster R, et al. Outcomes of autologous chondrocyte implantation in study of the treatment of articular repair (STAR) patients with osteochondritis dissecans. Am J Sports Med 2012;40(9):2015–22.

Management and Surgical Options for Articular Defects in the Shoulder

Bryan M. Saltzman, MD, Timothy Leroux, MD,
Brian J. Cole, MD, MBA*

KEYWORDS

- Shoulder • Glenohumeral • Chondral • Cartilage • Defects • Articular
- Autologous chondrocyte implantation • Osteochondral autograft

KEY POINTS

- The natural history of isolated, full-thickness chondral lesions of the glenohumeral joint is less clear than those of the knee or ankle.
- Often, the diagnosis can be difficult to make clinically because of vague, nonlocalized complaints, and a history and physical examination similar to other common shoulder pathologies.
- It is imperative that the surgeon obtain as much information as possible from the clinical evaluation so as to avoid treatment of an incidental, truly asymptomatic lesion.
- No firm consensus exists as of yet on the most appropriate operative treatment options for glenohumeral focal articular defects.
- Possible treatment measures include arthroscopic debridement, microfracture, autologous chondrocyte implantation, osteochondral allograft, and osteochondral autograft transfer, as well as biologic resurfacing or metallic replacement.

INTRODUCTION

Isolated, full-thickness chondral lesions of the glenohumeral joint are a significant pathology encountered by laborers, athletes, and the elderly.[1] They may be a result of genetic and/or degenerative changes to the joint, posttraumatic lesions, postoperative changes, loose bodies, osteonecrosis (iatrogenic, corticosteroid or alcohol use), shoulder instability or microinstability, inflammatory arthritis, osteoarthritis, infection, intra-articular pain pump placement, rotator cuff arthropathy, or osteochondritis dissecans.[2–4] The incidence of 5% to 17%[5] is less common than the knee joint, likely

Disclosure: See last page of article.
Department of Orthopedic Surgery, Rush University Medical Center, 1611 West Harrison Street, Suite 300, Chicago, IL 60612, USA
* Corresponding author.
E-mail address: brian.cole@rushortho.com

related to weight bearing and impact loading that is less in the shoulder joint. This is probably why many are well-tolerated and asymptomatic.[6] Diagnosis of full-thickness chondral defects can be challenging, and the outcomes following nonoperative and operative treatment less predictable.[2] Additionally, the natural history of full-thickness chondral lesions in the shoulder is less clear than those of the knee or ankle.[7]

The management of focal chondral lesions of the glenoid or humerus remains challenging.[8,9] These defects have a limited capacity to heal because of a lack of direct vascular supply and direct access to undifferentiated, pluripotent cells to assist with native healing capacity.[10] Thus, many treatment options have been refined to provide pain relief, create reparative tissue, or restore the articular surface.[8] Although shoulder arthroplasty is a reliable option for those with more diffuse degenerative changes, it can impose significant, debilitating activity restrictions for a younger individual and includes a limited implant life span. Joint-preserving procedures are therefore particularly important to identify for those young patients with focal cartilage defects with continued pain and decreased function.

CLASSIFICATION

No specific classification scheme pertains to articular lesions in the shoulder; as such, the Outerbridge system,[11] as is used to describe lesions in the knee, is conventionally used for the glenohumeral joint as well. In this, Grade 0 refers to normal cartilage, grade I is softening of the articular cartilage, grade II involves fibrillation of half the depth of the articular surface, grade III involves fissuring of more than half of the articular surface depth, and finally grade IV is full-thickness cartilage loss to the subchondral bone. Descriptive characteristics are otherwise pertinent, including location (humerus or glenoid), position (peripheral or central), size, depth, and degree of containment.

GLENOHUMERAL ARTICULAR ANATOMY

The anatomy of the glenohumeral joint can make evaluation and treatment of articular defects difficult. The mean articular depth of the glenoid fossa cartilage is 1.88 mm and that of the humerus cartilage is 1.24 mm.[12] The glenoid articular cartilage is thickest along the periphery and tapers toward the bare area in the center where no cartilage is present. By contrast, the humeral head chondral surface is thickest in the center (at approximately 1.2–1.3 mm thick) and thins to less than 1 mm at the periphery.[13] Knowledge of these characteristics is important when considering on patient imaging or arthroscopic evaluation whether a defect in the cartilage is present, or if it is just the native patient anatomy. In addition, the geometry of the glenohumeral joint is such that the glenoid radius of curvature is within 2 to 3 mm of the humeral head so that they remain relatively congruent with the interposed chondral surfaces and labral rim.[3] Glenoid version (1.5° retroversion) and inclination (4.2° superiorly) are important to consider for as well for approaching the joint surgically.[14]

HISTORY AND PHYSICAL EXAMINATION

A thorough history should be obtained in any patient presenting to the office with shoulder pain and concern for the etiology being an articular cartilage defect. Often the diagnosis can be difficult to make clinically because of vague, nonlocalized complaints and a history and physical examination similar to other common shoulder pathologies.[7] Because of the complex nature of the shoulder joint anatomy, careful consideration must be entertained for additional pathology to the rotator cuff, acromioclavicular joint, biceps, labrum, or capsule that may otherwise be the root of the patient's complaints. Not infrequently, intra-articular cartilage injury may be an incidental finding when another pathology is truly causing symptoms.

Traumatic events to the shoulder, including previous fractures, subluxations, or dislocations, should be investigated.[15] It is important to question the patient on prior surgical intervention on the glenohumeral joint; it can be very helpful to obtain prior operative reports and intraoperative imaging as well to review. It is imperative to note the nature and onset of symptoms as well as the progression of symptoms.[3] The quality of the patient's pain should be elucidated, as pain due to chondral defects are often dull and achy but with exacerbation by increased use. Sleep is also often affected.[15] Patients may additionally complain of mechanical symptoms, such as swelling, catching, and locking, in addition to a deep, activity-related pain as is also true for the knee joint.[1,15] The patient's age, current and desired activity level, and expectations/goals of treatment should be elucidated as well before discussing any potential therapeutic options.[3]

It is imperative that the surgeon obtain as much information as possible from the clinical evaluation so as to avoid treatment of an incidental, truly asymptomatic lesion. Physical examination should ensue as for any shoulder evaluation, including a documentation of passive and active range of motion, neurologic, and strength testing of the rotator cuff. The latter is pertinent given the reported increased incidence of articular cartilage injury in the presence of rotator cuff deficiency.[16] All examination findings should be compared with the contralateral "healthy" shoulder. Previous surgical scars should be documented. The presence of crepitus with motion may be indicative of an irregular joint surface and the possibility of chondral injury, whereas pain with compressive loads applied to the glenohumeral joint can additionally indicate the presence of an articular defect.[15] Special shoulder-specific tests should be performed to elicit any findings of concomitant pathology.[3] Unlike patients with osteoarthritis, these patients typically do not have significant limitations in motion.

IMAGING

The first-line imaging should always include plain radiographs of the glenohumeral joint, including a true anteroposterior view, scapular-Y, and axillary view to assess for any obvious osteophyte formation, subchondral sclerosis or cysts, or additional lucencies within the bone along the joint. The degree of joint space narrowing should be assessed.[15] The Stryker notch view and West Point view are helpful in evaluating Hill-Sachs lesions and glenoid bone loss, respectively, in a patient with history of instability.[17]

MRI provides the best evaluation of the chondral surface and surrounding soft tissues. It thus also allows for assessment of concomitant musculotendinous or labral pathology. The finding of a focal cartilage defect on the articular surface of the humeral head is often overlooked on MRI,[18] with rates as high as 45% for grade IV defects[19] due to the relatively thin cartilage in the shoulder. Standard sequences to evaluate articular cartilage include a T2-weighted image with or without fat suppression, and a T1-weighted fat-suppressed cartilage-sensitive sequence (ie, spoiled gradient-recalled echo or fast spin echo), which can demonstrate chondral fissuring, delamination, and focal loss.[20,21] Additionally, quantitative and semiquantitative techniques including delayed gadolinium-enhanced MRI of cartilage (dGEMRIC), T1rho, T2*, and T2 mapping techniques exist to better evaluate the composition of articular cartilage.[22] Subchondral bone marrow edema at the site of focal articular defects implies a possible traumatic origin to the injury, or may be suggestive of a full-thickness defect if the diagnosis is not clear.[18] Traumatic humeral head cartilage defects may be found medial to the expected location of a typical Hill-Sachs lesion, potentially due to shearing or compression from the undersurface of the acromion.[18]

Computed tomography (CT) imaging is helpful to evaluate glenohumeral joint alignment, glenoid bone loss, and version for those patients who may be indicated for osteochondral grafting to treat an articular defect.

NONOPERATIVE TREATMENT

Typically, the initial treatment of glenohumeral chondral disease is nonsurgical. This is similar to what is performed to relieve symptoms in other joints, and includes a trial of activity modification, physical therapy, oral nonsteroidal anti-inflammatory medications, and corticosteroid injections.[23] Physical therapy should focus on scapulothoracic and glenohumeral strengthening, stretching, and range of motion improvement.[3] Glenohumeral injection can be diagnostic as well as therapeutic when injected with lidocaine.[3]

BASIC SCIENCE RESEARCH

Few basic science efforts have evaluated the management of focal articular defects in the glenohumeral joint. Van Thiel and colleagues[24] evaluated the use of autologous matrix-induced chondrogenesis (AMIC) in rabbit glenohumeral cartilage defect models. AMIC involves use of a collagen I/III matrix with microfracture to promote the formation of nativelike cartilage architecture. In the 12 rabbit models, no statistically significant differences in micro-CT–determined total cartilage volume or average cartilage thickness were present in in those shoulders treated with microfracture alone, microfracture and AMIC, or control. However, a trend existed toward increased defect fill and thickness in the microfracture and AMIC groups.

Wang and colleagues[25] developed a rabbit shoulder animal model to study glenoid cartilage repair strategies and chondral healing. The investigators compared 45 rabbits in 3 groups: untreated glenoid articular surface defects, microfracture, and microfracture plus type I/III collagen scaffold (AMIC). At 32 weeks after surgery, the investigators demonstrated increased fibrous tissue deposition via micro-CT and a more hyalinelike histologic repair tissue with microfracture alone, whereas additional improvements with AMIC were seen only with MRI signal findings.

PALLIATIVE, REPARATIVE, AND RESTORATIVE SURGICAL OPTIONS

No firm consensus exists as of yet on the most appropriate operative treatment options for glenohumeral focal articular defects. Importantly, the presence of symptoms, not just that an articular defect exists, is what must guide the decision to intervene. Inappropriate surgical candidates include those tumors or infection of the glenohumeral joint, systemic cartilage disease, or inflammatory arthropathy.

Treatment measures may be palliative, reparative, restorative, or reconstructive.[24] Virtually all cartilage restoration options used in the knee can be applied to the shoulder as well.[20] Given the level of activity in these patients, joint-sparing surgery is preferred when nonoperative modalities fail. Nonarthroplasty options for active, young patients include debridement alone or with microfracture (with or without augmentation strategies), autologous chondrocyte implantation, and osteochondral transplantation. Indications are less well defined than in the knee joint, as the shoulder tolerates cartilage pathology better as a result of the relatively load-sparing nature of the joint and its wide arc of motion.[1] One must take into consideration the patient's defect location, size, depth, and containment, and the presence of any concurrent pathology that should be addressed at the time of intervention (**Table 1**).[3]

Gross and colleagues[26] reported that satisfaction rates are high in the literature (ranging from 66%–100%) for each of these procedures. The morbidity of the procedure must be considered in the decision-making process. Positive prognostic factors for this genre of intervention include lesion size less than 2 cm^2, unipolar lesions, less advanced lesions, and isolated lesions of the humerus. Negative prognostic variables included lesions greater than 2 cm^2, bipolar lesions, and prior surgical intervention.[26]

Arthroscopic Debridement

Palliative treatment with arthroscopic debridement, lavage, and loose body removal provides a relatively low morbidity procedure that does not burn bridges with future cartilage restoration procedures. At the very least, initial arthroscopic evaluation may provide a diagnostic assessment for the presence of chondral lesions to adequately stage and size the defect and determine the need for future intervention.[15] Its role in management specifically for chondral defects of the shoulder is limited in the literature, despite several studies indicating successful outcomes when used in the setting of generalized osteoarthritis.

Typical components of this procedure include removal of loose bodies, synovectomy, capsular release for motion loss, and subacromial decompression if felt to be a component of the patient's symptoms. The removal of chondral flaps with arthroscopic curettes and motorized shavers may help decrease mechanical symptoms.[3] It can be biomechanically beneficial as well to create a stable, vertical transition zone between full-thickness cartilage defects and the surrounding normal cartilage.[3]

Cameron and colleagues[19] reported on the results of 61 patients (mean age, 49.5 years) who underwent arthroscopic debridement with or without capsular release with grade IV articular lesions of the glenohumeral joint. Of the 45 patients with minimum 2-year follow-up, the mean patient satisfaction score improved significantly from 0.67 to 6.28 (P<.0001) with 87% of patients indicating that they would have the surgery performed again. Significant improvements in patient pain and function were noted in 88% of all patients (P<.0001) despite workers' compensation patients having inferior results. The onset of pain relief was noted for most patients by 5 weeks postoperative, and lasted for more than 28 months. The investigators found an association with return of pain and procedural failure for lesions larger than 2 cm^2.

Kerr and McCarty[27] reported on the outcomes of patients with either unipolar or bipolar chondral defects of the shoulder who received arthroscopic debridement. Most of these patients, however, had concurrent procedures during the debridement (16 of 19 patients including 36% with capsular release), including 2 with microfracture. Ultimately, patients at 28 months postoperative had significant pain relief (88%) and 87% were satisfied with the procedure. The investigators noted that patients with unipolar lesions had superior outcomes, and outcomes worsened with articular defect size greater than 2 × 2 cm^2.

Microfracture

Although much more commonly reported in the knee because of its ease as a first-line treatment option with low surgical morbidity and successful clinical outcomes,[1] the use of microfracture in the glenohumeral joint provides an option for isolated full-thickness cartilage defects that is minimally invasive, technically nondemanding, and potentially fruitful. Microfracture creates a channel to the underlying marrow to

Table 1
Summary of reparative and restorative interventions for chondral defects in the glenohumeral joint

Surgical Intervention	Indications	Contraindications	Technical Pearls	Rehabilitation
Microfracture	• Failed conservative management • Potential first-line option for small defects • Borrowed from knee literature: size <2 cm^2, BMI <30 kg/m^2, age <45 y, symptoms >12 mo • Unipolar • Congruent glenohumeral joint	• Generalized DJD • Hyperlaxity • Bipolar lesions • Presence of concomitant intra-articular pathology (unless concurrently addressed) • Uncontained lesions • Partial-thickness lesions • Chondral lesions with associated relevant bony defects • Violated subchondral plate • Relatively larger or bipolar lesions	• Beach chair or lateral decubitus • Careful consideration for anterior portal placement to facilitate perpendicular access to defect (more lateral for glenoid lesions, more medial for humeral lesions) • Diagnostic arthroscopy and concurrent procedures performed first • Be certain the cartilage defect is contained • Curette or shaver to create stable vertical walls and debride calcified cartilage layer • 30° or 90° awl or PowerPick to create microfracture holes perpendicular to the joint	• CPM vs no CPM • Gentle WBAT after surgery • Phase I: protective passive ROM weeks 0–8 • Phase II – active ROM and strengthening weeks 9–14 • Phase III – return to sport weeks 15–17 • No heavy lifting for 3 mo • Full activity allowed at 4 mo • No overhead athletic competition for 6 mo

| Augmented microfracture (ie, micronized allogeneic cartilage matrix implantation) | (As for microfracture alone) | • Best to have positioned in lateral decubitus to avoid gravity effects on implantation
• Turn off arthroscopic fluid and suction joint dry
• Prepare BioCartilage mixture with PRP
• Thin layer of fibrin glue in the prepared, dried defect bed
• Introduce BioCartilage mixture paste onto the defect so that it is slightly recessed when compared with surrounding chondral margins
• Freer elevator can be used to smooth over the surface of the BioCartilage, and a thin layer of fibrin glue is used to seal over the top of this and the neighboring cartilage | • Sling for 4–6 wk with removal for active and active-assisted ROM activities
• Otherwise as for microfracture alone |

(continued on next page)

Table 1
(continued)

Surgical Intervention	Indications	Contraindications	Technical Pearls	Rehabilitation
Autologous chondrocyte implantation (ACI)	• Young adult (<40 y old) • Isolated lesion • Large lesion not amenable to OATS • Full-thickness defect • Smaller, contained superficial defects	• Relevant subchondral bone edema	• Cartilage biopsy (harvest) site either at the intercondylar notch of the knee, or at healthy cartilage near the shoulder defect • Open approach (deltopectoral) • Obtain hemostasis at the base of the defect • Debride the defect but do not violate the subchondral bone plate • Periosteal patch harvest from medial tibia, or instead a type I/III collagen-based membrane matrix can be used • Fibrin glue along the periphery of the periosteal patch	• CPM machine suggested, 6–8 h daily • At 4 wk, 90° elevation and 20° ER active-assisted motion allowed • At 6 wk, 140° elevation and 40° ER active-assisted motion allowed • At 12 wk, no restrictions • Questionable return to over-head throwing

Procedure	Indications	Technique	Rehabilitation
Osteochondral autograft transfer	• Young patients • As a first-line treatment • Relatively smaller (10–20 mm diameter) defect sizes for autografting are proposed • Combined cartilage and bone loss (osteochondral injury)	• Open, open-assist arthroscopic, or all-arthroscopic means • Autografting harvest site is the ipsilateral sulcus of the lateral femoral condyle • Press-fit technique for graft to recipient site • Bio-Compression screw for backup fixation	• Sling initially postoperative (<1 wk) • Active-assisted and passive ROM exercises POD#1 • At 3 wk, active ROM allowed • At 5 wk, strengthening exercises introduced • At 6 mo, return to overhead sport
Osteochondral allograft	• Young patients • As a first-line treatment • Larger, full-thickness defects • Combined cartilage and bone loss (osteochondral injury)	• Open, open-assist arthroscopic, or all-arthroscopic means • Press-fit technique for graft to recipient site • Bio-Compression screw for backup fixation	• Sling initially postoperative (<1 wk) • Active-assisted and passive ROM exercises POD#1 • At 3 wk, active ROM allowed • At 5 wk, strengthening exercises introduced • At 6 mo, return to overhead sport

Abbreviations: BMI, body mass index; CPM, continuous passive motion; DJD, degenerative joint disease; ER, external rotation; OATS, osteochondral autograft transfer system; POD, postoperative day; PRP, platelet-rich plasma; ROM, range of motion; WBAT, weight bearing as tolerated.

encourage chondral resurfacing with fibrocartilage at the site of a focal defect through an introduction of mesenchymal stem cells, growth factors, fibrin, and platelets.[28] Given that the scapula and humerus have excellent vascular supply, it would seem plausible that the glenohumeral joint could expect similar success to the knee with microfracture surgery.[7] It appears to be a viable option for both acute and chronic articular cartilage lesions,[9] and its use avoids the harvest site morbidity of autografting procedures for chondral defect repair yet does not compromise the surgeon's performance of more aggressive subsequent procedures.[3]

There is no formal defect size limit for microfracture, as is quoted consistently through the knee literature, due to the relative paucity of microfracture literature in the glenohumeral joint.[1] However, smaller lesion size is preferred for treatment.[9] Patients should have a focal, symptomatic lesion that has failed conservative management, and the joint should be congruent. From the literature of microfracture use in the knee, considerations of patient chondral defect size (<2 cm^2), age (<45 years), body mass index (<30 kg/m^2), and symptom duration (>12 months) are helpful to identify a patient who will maximally benefit from the intervention.[29]

Absolute contraindications include the presence of generalized degenerative joint osteoarthritis, high-grade ligamentous laxity, partial-thickness lesions or lesions associated with large bony defects, and subchondral plate violation.[1,9] Relative contraindications included lesions of larger size or those with untreated bipolar counterparts,[15] the latter of which may be better treated with glenoid microfracture but biologic restorative means (such as osteochondral allografting) of the humerus.[15] Microfracture should additionally not be performed in isolation if intervention is needed to address concomitant rotator cuff injury, labral or biceps disease, or shoulder instability, in which repeated postoperative subluxations/dislocations may affect the healing capacity from microfracture (see **Table 1**).[1,15]

With the surgical technique, the patient can be placed either in beach chair or lateral decubitus position based on surgeon preference. A standard posterior portal is used; the position of the anterior working portal is judged based on the location of the chondral defect being addressed so that a more direct, perpendicular route is attainable to the lesion.[1] That is, a more lateral position of the anterior portal will be beneficial to work at the anterosuperior glenoid, whereas a more inferior portal can help reach a defect in the inferior glenoid. Conversely, a more medial position for the portal will benefit access to the humerus, and internal and external rotation of the head will help enable the approach. A posterior 7-o'clock portal may allow easier access to the posterior glenoid.[1]

After diagnostic arthroscopy, any additional concurrent pathology should be addressed first so as to maintain clarity in visualization for these concomitant interventions that can be lost after microfracture.[1] It is necessary to confirm containment of the chondral defect before proceeding.[1] Standard procedure for microfracture is then performed as in other joints throughout the body: debridement with an arthroscopic shaver, ring curette, or basket forceps can ensure proper removal of overlying calcified cartilage.[1] A combination of arthroscopic elevator, shaver, and curette can be used to create stable vertical walls circumferentially to facilitate the fibrous clot formation after microfracture. The calcified cartilage layer is debrided in its entirety, typically with an arthroscopic curette or the shaver run in forward or reverse direction, with confirmation through punctate bleeding in the bone base.[9] As the concavity of the glenoid can make it difficult to place the microfracture awl tip perpendicular to its surface, it is suggested to use a 90° awl for superior positioning. The 30° awl is often more appropriate for the humeral head, which is typically easier to access.[1] The PowerPick instrumentation can otherwise be used if preferred.[4]

Augmentation strategies including micronized allogeneic cartilage matrix (Bio-Cartilage) implantation can be considered in an attempt to restore the glenohumeral joint surface with a more hyaline-type cartilage as opposed to the fibrocartilage generated from microfracture alone.[4] When this is deemed appropriate, the arthroscopic pump is shut off and the joint fluid suctioned to thoroughly dry the defect site. The Bio-Cartilage mixture paste is mixed with platelet-rich plasma (PRP) and placed over a thin layer of fibrin glue to fill the defect almost to the level of the surrounding healthy cartilage. Another layer of fibrin glue is placed over the top of the smoothed BioCartilage surface.[4]

Well-defined rehabilitative protocols following microfracture of the shoulder joint are limited. The shoulder differs from the knee in terms of its decreased joint volume and synovial lining, and increased range of motion; thus, some investigators[1] have advocated against use of continuous passive motion (CPM) machines, as patients can often move their shoulder appropriately after surgery to stimulate synovial fluid production. As the shoulder is not a load-bearing joint, patients can bear weight as tolerated, with avoidance of heavy overhead lifting and competitive overhead athletics for 3 and 6 months, respectively.[1]

Hensley and Sum[30] provide a detailed postoperative rehabilitation protocol including a 3-phase approach. Phase I includes protective passive range of motion from 0 to 8 weeks postoperatively. Phase II includes active range of motion and strengthening from 9 to 14 weeks postoperatively. Phase III is a return to sport phase from weeks 15 to 17 postoperatively, with a focus on advanced strengthening, control, and introduction of resistance activities while maintaining and improving shoulder motion.

Siebold and colleagues[31] reported on 5 patients who underwent a combination of open microfracture and periosteal flap for the treatment of focal full-thickness humeral head chondral lesions. Three of the patients had undergone instability treatment previously, and 2 again at the time of microfracture surgery. Mean patient age was 32 years, and mean lesion size was 311 mm^2. Patients had significant improvements at a mean follow-up of 25.8 months in Constant score (43.4% to 81.8%) and pain reduction (to 18.6 points). Second-look arthroscopy in 3 patients at a mean 8 months postoperative demonstrated significantly reduced chondral lesion sizes.

Snow and Funk[7] evaluated 8 patients who underwent arthroscopic microfracture to treat full-thickness chondral lesions smaller than 4 cm^2. The mean age was 37 years, and 7 patients (87.5%) underwent concurrent procedures. Five of the treated defects were at the humeral head, and the remaining 3 at the glenoid. The investigators ultimately saw significant improvements in Constant and Oxford scores, with no complications. Two second-look arthroscopic surgeries demonstrated good lesion filling with fibrocartilage.

Millett and colleagues[9] described the results of microfracture in 30 patients (31 shoulders), including 6 patients with bipolar lesion treatment, 13 with glenoid defect treatment, and 12 with humeral head microfracture. Although the investigators reported a failure rate of 19% (6 of 31 shoulders), at a mean 47 months of follow-up, pain scores, patient ability to work, and performance of activities of daily living and sport activities all significantly improved. The mean American Shoulder and Elbow Surgeons (ASES) score improved by 20 points as well, and patients expressed a mean satisfaction of 7.6 of 10. The investigators found the greatest significance in improvement for those patients with isolated humeral head lesions that received treatment; a negative correlation was found between lesion size and ASES improvement, and patients with bipolar treated lesions were least improved.

Slabaugh and colleagues[1] described a case report of a patient in his early 40s with a 10-year history of right shoulder pain who was successfully treated with microfracture of a 25 × 25-mm focal chondral defect on the humeral head. He regained full shoulder motion, complete satisfaction, and full strength postoperatively.

Frank and colleagues[5] reported on 17 shoulders in 16 patients who underwent microfracture of the glenoid (n = 6), humerus (n = 10), and both surfaces (n = 1) at a mean follow-up of 27.8 months. The mean patient age was 37 years, with average humeral and glenoid defect sizes of 5.07 cm² and 1.66 cm², respectively. The investigators reported failure (by means of subsequent surgical intervention) in 3 patients. The investigators reported significant improvements in visual analog scale (VAS) pain scores (5.6–1.9), Simple Shoulder Test score (5.7–10.3), and ASES score (44.3–86.3). They reported that 12 patients (92.3%) said they would have the procedure performed again.

Hensley and Sum[30] reported on a 46-year-old male powerlifter with grade IV chondral lesions of the humeral head and articular surface of the superior glenoid rim measuring 2 to 3 cm in diameter each. He underwent microfracture of both defects with concurrent debridement of a type I superior labral tear from anterior to posterior (SLAP) and subacromial decompression. The patient at 2 years postoperatively was very satisfied with his outcome, with substantial improvements in all QuickDASH subscores and a return to lifting, although at much lower weight quantities (**Table 2**).

Autologous Chondrocyte Implantation

At present, there is not definitive evidence for the use of autologous chondrocyte implantation (ACI) in the shoulder, as the literature is much more scarce than is present for the knee joint. Some investigators believe it to be a promising avenue for treatment, at least in part because of the low loads experienced by the joint. The autologous chondrocytes produce anabolic growth factors to promote cell survival and induce chondrocyte proliferation at the site of implantation; however, concerns exist for its use because of the relatively high levels of shear stress during shoulder rotational motions, such as overhead throwing, which could affect the integrity of the ACI procedure.[8] Considering the positive results demonstrated in the use of ACI for articular defects in the knee, however, its use in the shoulder has begun to be evaluated.

The optimal indication is for a contained, unipolar, superficial, or surface defect devoid of subchondral bone involvement/edema in the humerus or glenoid in a relatively young patient (age <40 years) who failed cartilage reparative techniques (ie, microfracture).[20,32] It otherwise may be implemented in larger lesions not amenable to osteochondral autograft transplantation or more superficial lesions in which violating the subchondral surface (as occurs with osteochondral grafting) is to be avoided. Potential morbidity may be introduced by the open approach required for the procedure, or the 2-step approach required to harvest and subsequently implant the chondrocytes (see **Table 1**).

Autologous cartilage can be harvested from the knee at the intercondylar notch, in the location of a typical notchplasty during anterior cruciate ligament reconstruction. ACI can be performed within 1 month thereafter.[8] Other sources have included at the location of macroscopic healthy cartilage near the defect site.[32] An open approach using the deltopectoral interval is most appropriate for surgical visualization and performance of the procedure. The articular edges of the defect are debrided to stable vertical walls, such as with a ringed curette, with careful hemostasis obtained at the base of the defect. The subchondral bone plate does not need to be violated with this debridement.

A periosteal patch can be harvested from the medial tibia just distal to the pes anserine, and sutured to the remaining cartilage using 6 to 0 Vicryl sutures with a small opening left for injection of the chondrocyte suspension.[8] A collagen I/III-based matrix membrane can be used instead of a periosteal flap to avoid donor site morbidity, excessive suturing, and the rate of graft hypertrophy.[33] Fibrin glue is used along the circumference of the periosteal patch to create a watertight seal. The suspension is injected, and the remaining defect sutured and sealed.

Some investigators have suggested use of CPM machine after this procedure for 6 to 8 hours daily with initial weight-bearing restrictions.[8] Active-assisted motion to 20° of external rotation and 90° of elevation is typically allowed at 4 weeks postoperative; this is increased to 40° and 140°, respectively, at 6 weeks postoperative. Restrictions are eliminated at 12 weeks postoperative for strengthening and range of motion. Return to overhead throwing activities is questionable.[8]

Only 2 published studies exist on the use of ACI in the shoulder. Romeo and colleagues[8] described a case report of a 16-year-old boy with a 2-year history of insidious-onset right shoulder pain related to throwing a baseball. After an outside surgeon had performed an arthroscopic subacromial decompression and thermal shrinkage, he began to develop increased mechanical symptoms in the subsequent months, and clinical evaluation suggested a posterosuperior labral tear. At the time of revision arthroscopic stabilization, the patient was noted to have a 3.3 × 1.5-cm full-thickness chondral defect in the anterosuperior humeral head. After this procedure, the patient had continued symptoms and was deemed appropriate for autologous cartilage harvest from the knee with subsequent ACI performance in the shoulder 1 month later. At 12 months postoperative, the patient demonstrated full and painless range of motion with no complaints of pain at rest.

Buchmann and colleagues[32] reported on 4 consecutive male patients (mean age, 29.3 ± 6.2 years) who underwent ACI for large symptomatic glenoid (1 measuring 2.0 cm^2) or humeral (3, measuring each 6.0 cm^2) full-thickness chondral defects. At a mean follow-up of 41.3 ± 24.9 months, all patients had satisfactory shoulder function with mean postoperative VAS scores of 0.3, mean unweighted Constant scores of 83.3 ± 9.9, and mean ASES index of 95.3 ± 8.1. Patients additionally underwent MRI, which indicated satisfactory coverage of the defect locations with signs of fibrocartilaginous repair tissue formation (see **Table 2**).

Osteochondral Autograft Transfer

Advantages of osteochondral autograft transfer include the ability to restore the glenohumeral architecture with a viable "organ" of live cartilage and bone through a single-stage procedure. It additionally provides the opportunity to achieve osseous integration while preserving the articular tidemark.[3] Disadvantages of osteochondral autograft include specifically donor site morbidity, and allograft as well as autografting risks dead space between circular grafts, graft integration, and the differing mechanical properties and geometry between the recipient and donor cartilage sites.[34]

Some investigators believe that osteochondral graftings are less appealing as an initial treatment option in young patients because of the destruction it requires to the healthy subchondral bone and lack of good salvage procedures should it fail.[8] It is typically used in the genre of anterior shoulder instability repair, for those shoulders with Hill-Sachs lesions caused by the impact of the posterolateral aspect of the humeral head on the anterior aspect of the glenoid at the time of dislocation, or in others with large, uncontained defects with subchondral bone loss.[20] Often, as with ACI, this is considered a second-line procedure after failed cartilage reparative techniques (ie, microfracture), but can be used as a first-line procedure.

The ideal osteochondral defect size for osteochondral autologous transplantation to the shoulder is between 10 and 20 mm in diameter or an area of 1.0 to 1.5 cm^2.[34]

Table 2
Clinical outcome studies on reparative and restorative treatments for glenohumeral chondral defects

Authors	Operative Treatment	Defect Location	Study Type/ Cohort Size	Patient Information	Clinical Outcomes
Slabaugh et al,[1] 2010	Microfracture	Humerus	Case report N = 1	• Early 40-something year old, 10-y history of shoulder pain, failed nonsurgical management • Lesion size: 25 × 25 mm	• 3/10 pain → 0/10 pain (on VAS scale) • ASES score 62 → 100 • Full ROM, strength • Complete satisfaction
Hensley et al,[30] 2011	Microfracture	Glenoid AND humerus	Case report N = 1	• 46 y-old male power lifter • Full-thickness humerus lesion, lesion of articulating surface of superior glenoid rim, both 2–3 cm in diameter • Concurrent SLAP debridement, SAD	• 2-y postoperative • QuickDASH sport 100 → 25; work 56.25 → 6.25; ADLs 40.9 → 4.5 • Minimal, intermittent stiffness • Very satisfied
Siebold et al,[31] 2003	Microfracture (+periosteal flap)	Humerus	Case series N = 5	• Grade IV defects, mean size 311 mm^2 (range, 225–400 mm^2) • Mean age, 32 y (range, 16–56 y) • Concurrent surgeries: posterior capsule shift (2), anchor removal (2), labral augmentation (1) • 3 with prior surgeries (open or arthroscopic Bankart repairs)	• Mean follow-up 25.8 mo • 3 patients with second-look scope at mean 8 mo, all with significantly reduced lesion sizes • Constant score significantly improved 43.4% → 81.8% • Pain reduced significantly to 18.6 points • Radiography and MRI showed progression of arthritis in 2 patients
Snow et al,[7] 2008	Microfracture	Glenoid OR humerus	Case series N = 8	• 6 men, 2 women • Mean age, 37 y (range, 27–55 y) • Lesion size <4 cm^2 • 1 isolated surgery, 7 with concurrent procedures (2 SAD, 2 capsular plication, 3 anterior stabilization) • 5 humeral head defects, 3 glenoid defects	• Mean follow-up of 15.4 mo (range, 12–27 mo) • Mean Constant score 43.88 → 90.25 (P<.005) • Mean Oxford score 25.75 → 17 (P<.005) • No complications • 2 second-look operations, both showed good filling with fibrocartilage

Millett et al,[9] 2009	Microfracture	Glenoid AND/OR humerus	Case series N = 31 shoulders (30 patients)	• 25 men, 5 women • Mean age, 43 y • 6 both humeral (mean 442 mm²) and glenoid (mean 273 mm²); 13 just glenoid (mean 137 mm²); 12 just humeral head (mean 422 mm²) • Concomitant procedures: 6 instability procedures, 10 SADs, 7 capsular releases or manipulations under anesthesia, 7 SLAP lesion debridements/repairs, 3 biceps releases	• Mean final follow-up, 47 mo • Mean pain scores 3.8 → 1.6 • Significant improvements in patients' ability to work, ADLs, sports activity ($P<.05$) • Painless use of involved arm improved ($P<.05$) • Mean ASES score improved by 20 points ($P<.05$) • Mean satisfaction 7.6 of 10 • No association between age/gender and outcomes • Greatest improvements when isolated lesion to humerus • Worst with bipolar lesions • Failure in 6 of 31 (19%): 3 shoulder replacements at mean 41 mo, 1 shoulder instability procedure, 1 biceps/instability, 1 unknown procedure
Frank et al,[5] 2010	Microfracture	Glenoid AND/OR humerus	Case series N = 17 shoulders (16 patients)	• Mean age 37.0 y (range, 18–55 y) • 7 men, 5 women in final analysis (2 lost to follow-up, 3 failures) • Average humeral defect size, 5.07 cm² (range, 1.0–7.84 cm²) • Average glenoid defect size, 1.66 cm² (range, 0.4–3.75 cm²)	• Mean 27.8-mo follow-up • Three failures (subsequent shoulder surgery) • Significant VAS pain improvement 5.6 → 1.4 ($P<.01$) • Significant Simple Shoulder Test improvement 5.7 → 10.3 ($P<.01$) • Significant ASES improvement (44.3 → 86.3) • 92.3% said they would have the procedure performed again

(continued on next page)

Table 2
(continued)

Authors	Operative Treatment	Defect Location	Study Type/ Cohort Size	Patient Information	Clinical Outcomes
Buchmann et al,[32] 2012	ACI	Glenoid OR humerus	Case series N = 4	• 4 men • Mean age, 29.3 ± 6.2 y • 3 humeral full-thickness defects (each 6.0 cm^2), 1 glenoid full-thickness defect (2.0 cm^2) • Humeral locations: anterior-superior, posterior-central, central • Glenoid location: posterior • Concomitant surgeries: 2 loose body extraction, 1 anchor extraction, 1 tenodesis of long head of biceps, 1 microfracture of anterior glenoid	• Final follow-up, mean 41.3 ± 24.9 mo • Mean VAS 0.3 of 10 • Mean unweighted Constant score 83.3 ± 9.9 • Mean ASES index 95.3 ± 8.1 • MRI with satisfactory defect coverage with signs of fibrocartilaginous repair tissue
Romeo et al,[8] 2002	ACI	Humerus	Case report N = 1	• 16 y old, 2-y history of shoulder pain, failed arthroscopic SAD and capsular thermal shrinkage • Lesion size: 33 × 15 mm	• At 12 mo, full ROM without pain • No further complaints, no pain at rest
Camp et al,[43] 2015	OA	Glenoid	Case report N = 1	• 25-y-old former multisport athlete • 6-y history of pain • 15-mm-diameter defect • Medial tibial plateau osteochondral allo- graft source	• At 1 y postoperative, subjective shoulder value score 40% → 99% • QuickDASH score 36 → 2 • ASES score 46 → 92 • Articular surface restoration maintained at 6-mo MRI

Study	Procedure	Location	Study design	Defect/Patient characteristics	Outcomes
Park et al,[35] 2006	OATS	Humerus	Case report N = 1	• 13-y-old boy • Defect on posterosuperior head, 9 mm • Harvest site, ipsilateral sulcus of the lateral femoral condyle • All arthroscopic	• At 5-mo postoperative, second-look arthroscopy demonstrated healed and covered with congruent hyaline cartilage • Final follow-up 31 mo, no symptoms and good functional results with radiographic resolution
Kircher et al,[38] 2009	OATS	Glenoid OR humerus	Case series N = 7	• Age range, 23.4–57.1 y (mean 43.1 y) • 6 men, 1 woman • Defects on anterocentral glenoid (1); central (3), posteromedial (1), posterocentral (1) and anterocentral (1) humerus • Mean 1.86 osteochondral cylinders used • Mean size of affected area 150 mm^2 • 4 isolated procedures; 3 with concurrent labral augmentation and capsular shift • Harvest site on ipsilateral knee	Note: The investigators reported outcomes at mean 32.6 mo (Scheibel et al,[34] 2004), where patients had significant increases in mean Constant score and MRI evidence of good osseointegration and congruent cartilage site in all but 1 patient • Mean final follow-up 8.75 y • 100% very satisfied • No reoperations • Mean Constant score 76.2 → 90.9 ($P = .018$) • Mean Lysholm score 100 → 99.3 • One patient had marginal decline in knee function • From first to final follow-up, 3 patients showed no change in pain but 3 showed an increase in their pain score ($P = .257$) • 100% increased level of ADLs ($P = .018$) • All but one with significant strength increase ($P = .028$) • All patients with increased OA classification at final follow-up • All but 1 patient with congruent joint surface on final MRI; all grafts fully integrated into surrounding bone

Abbreviations: ACI, autologous chondrocyte implantation; ADL, activities of daily living; ASES, American Shoulder and Elbow Surgeons; OA, osteochondral allograft; OATS, osteochondral autograft transplantation system; ROM, range of motion; SAD, subacromial decompression; SLAP, superior labral tear from anterior to posterior; VAS, visual analog scale.

Osteochondritis dissecans of the humeral head, although an uncommon disorder in young patients, is another pathology that may warrant osteochondral transplantation. This involves a localized involvement of part of the subchondral bone and overlying articular cartilage that results in separation of the two and a resultant defect in the chondral surface (see **Table 1**).[35]

The procedure can be performed through an open approach, or by all-arthroscopic means.[36] With autografting, a donor plug can be harvested through an open approach from the lateral trochlea of the knee just proximal to the sulcus terminalis. Osteoarticular bone is reamed at the recipient site, to match the sized core of osteochondral graft. Fixation can be achieved through press-fitting, partially threaded cancellous screws, or headless compression screws.[37]

Postoperative rehabilitation varies after allograft or autograft transplantation. Sling use for the first week after surgery is advised by some investigators, with active-assisted and passive range of motion exercises allowed as soon as postoperative day 1. At 3 weeks postoperative, active range of motion is initiated, and strengthening exercises are introduced at 5 weeks from surgery. Return to overhead sport may be feasible at 6 months from the date of surgery.

Park and colleagues[35] performed an arthroscopic osteochondral autograft transfer in treatment of an osteochondral defect of the humeral head of a 13-year-old boy with an osteochondral lesion measuring 9 mm in diameter. The investigators obtained a bony graft from the ipsilateral sulcus of the lateral femoral condyle, and transplanted the tissue through arthroscopic means to the posterosuperior defect site. At a second-look arthroscopic surgery 5 months postoperative, the defects at the harvest site and pathologic site were completely healed and covered with congruent articular hyaline cartilage. With final 31-month follow-up, the patient had no symptoms and good functional results, with radiographic resolution of the defect.

Scheibel and colleagues[34] reported on 8 patients at medium-term follow-up of 32.6 months after osteochondral autologous transplantation to the humerus and/or glenoid. The mean patient age was 43.1 years. The patients had a mean defect size of 150 mm^2. Four patients underwent concurrent procedures at the time of the index intervention (labral augmentation and capsular shift). The investigators reported significant improvements in the mean Constant score, with MRI demonstrating good osseointegration of the osteochondral plugs and congruent articular surface at the site of transplantation for all but 1 patient. Macroscopic appearance in 2 patients who underwent second-look arthroscopy showed an intact surface as well. Kircher and colleagues[38] reported on 7 of the aforementioned patients (6 humeral, 1 glenoid) at a mean long-term follow-up of 8.75 years as well. Patients significantly improved in terms of mean Constant score and Lysholm score, although a significant progress of osteoarthritic changes was present from preoperative to final follow-up, unrelated to the defect size, number of cylinder use, or the Constant score. Postoperative imaging demonstrated congruent joint surfaces at the defect in all but 1 patient, with full bony integration of all osteochondral grafts. Ultimately, the investigators suggested a satisfactory outcome over a long follow-up period from the surgery with very good subjective and objective findings.

Osteochondral Allograft

The use of osteochondral allografts to address chondral articular defects in the knee has been well established,[39] but its utility in the shoulder has been evaluated only more recently. The goal with osteochondral grafting is to recreate the congruency of the articular surface (**Fig. 1**).[3] It requires a thorough appreciation for the morphology of

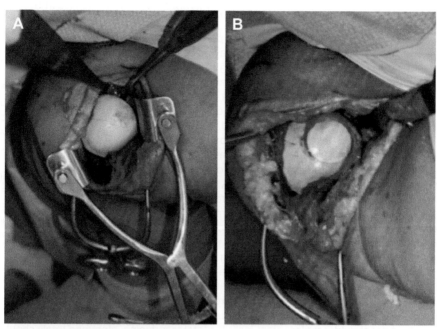

Fig. 1. (*A*) Symptomatic chondral lesion in a 30-year-old active man having failed prior arthroscopic debridement. (*B*) Image of osteochondral allograft (OA) plug in place of defect in same 30-year-old man.

the native glenohumeral joint to ensure proper placement and sizing.[40] Concern exists at the glenoid as to whether reaming may cause a cortical blowout, and thus whether adequate depth of reaming can occur to provide a stable press-fit of an osteochondral graft. Accommodation of graft size decreases significantly as the reaming depth is increased above 4 mm.[41]

The procedure is performed similarly to the aforementioned approach for osteo-chondral autografting. The source of osteochondral allografts can be fresh or fresh-frozen, and include femoral head allograft or humeral head allograft sources. Recent data suggest that the talar dome has a high degree of surface congruency when compared with the humeral head, with maximal graft sizes of 30 × 10 mm; this may be a potential future source option as an alternative to a size-matched humeral head allograft.[42] Postoperative rehabilitation is similar to the aforementioned protocol recommendations for osteochondral autografting.

Humeral head osteochondral allograft transplantation has been evaluated in terms of large Hill-Sachs lesions due to instability with significant improvements in shoulder motion and ASES scores as far as 1-year postoperatively, and with high rates of re-turn to work and satisfaction despite substantial complication and reoperation rates.[37] Camp and colleagues[43] reported the use in a 25-year-old male former multi-sport athlete of a tibial osteochondral allograft to restore a large glenoid osteochon-dral defect. The investigators had a successful result at 1-year postoperative with significant improvements in the patient's QuickDASH score (from 36 to 2), subjective shoulder value (from 40% to 99%), and ASES score (from 46 to 92). MRI demon-strated maintained congruity of the articular surface at 6 months postoperative (see **Table 2**).

BIOLOGIC RESURFACING AND RECONSTRUCTIVE SURGICAL OPTIONS

For those young patients with advanced bipolar lesions not amenable to reparative or restorative options, biologic resurfacing may be used. This refers to the use of soft tissue interposition within the joint, including fascia lata, allograft tendon, periosteum, porcine small intestine submucosa, anterior shoulder capsule, or allograft meniscus,[20,44] to biologically resurface the glenoid with either biologic or nonbiologic resurfacing of the humeral head. The procedure is most often performed in association with hemiarthroplasty of the humeral head.[45] The use of this technology is to bridge the treatment gap for this demographic of patients who are not yet candidates for total shoulder arthroplasty. The goal is thus to avoid the complications of glenoid component loosening and morbidity of revision procedures for young, typically high-demand patients who can be seen with arthroplasty surgery.[6] Few clinical studies have evaluated these techniques, but results are generally positive.[23,44,46–48]

Additional reconstructive efforts with metallic replacement means are typically reserved for the more diffuse, osteoarthritic shoulder rather than for the management of a focal articular defect. However, these may be required for use as salvage options when failure has occurred, or in the setting of bipolar disease in which the aforementioned options are less appropriate. These include open lateral meniscal allograft or dermal patch resurfacing, the glenoid ream-and-run procedure with humeral head implant resurfacing, and total shoulder arthroplasty.[49] Partial shoulder arthroplasty options include inlay arthroplasty, hemiresurfacing, and stemmed hemiarthroplasty,[50] whereas total shoulder replacement includes total resurfacing, stemmed totals shoulder arthroplasty, and reverse shoulder arthroplasty. Total shoulder arthroplasty remains an option for older patients with more diffuse, symptomatic cartilage disease, but imposes significant limitations on the younger patient with a more focal articular defect. These interventions remain outside of the scope of this review article, but their outcomes in the young adult are well described in the literature.[3]

FUTURE DIRECTIONS: PLATELET-RICH PLASMA?

PRP has shown greater promise as an emerging biological therapy for the treatment of chondral injury and cartilage repair efforts in the knee because it provides numerous bioactive growth factors at the site of application.[51] PRP increases chondrocyte and mesenchymal stem cell proliferation, proteoglycan deposition, and type II collagen deposition, and it has been used as an independent intra-articular injection, or as an adjunct to concomitant surgical management in the knee (ie, microfracture surgery, graft/scaffold/implant insertion).[52] It has also been described in clinic use for Achilles tendon rupture, chronic rotator cuff tendinopathy or tearing, muscle injury, chronic tendinosis, and meniscal repair.[53] The use of PRP in the glenohumeral joint for articular defects has not yet been evaluated in the literature, however.

OVERALL KEY PRINCIPLES IN TREATMENT

Gross and colleagues[26] suggested 5 key principles to guide treatment of focal articular defects of the glenohumeral joint that hold true when considering the most recent literature updates: (1) arthroscopic debridement alone should be considered when a lesion is encountered incidentally; (2) biologic resurfacing should be considered when lesions are bipolar; (3) osteoarticular graft or resurfacing should be considered when the lesion involves bone loss; (4) microfracture and osteochondral autograft transfer system (OATS) should be considered when the lesion is small; and (5) ACI or osteochondral allograft (OA) should be considered when the lesion is large.

CONCLUDING THOUGHTS

Articular cartilage defects in the glenohumeral joint remain a challenging pathology for the treating orthopedic surgeon. A thorough workup of the patient needs to be performed to confirm a symptomatic defect. The patient's articular defect characteristics, symptoms, and activity level all must be taken into consideration when developing a treatment plan for this complex problem.

Gross and colleagues[26] conducted a systematic review of clinical outcomes after many of the aforementioned cartilage restorative and reparative procedures in the glenohumeral joint. In their synthesis of the data, they identified that most studies reported favorable results, but the evidence available for the use of these procedures is considered "very low" and "any estimate of effect is very uncertain." The investigators reported, however, that all of these studies are observational, retrospective case series without control groups.

These investigators highlighted how high-quality evidence is clearly lacking for any of these procedures in the glenohumeral joint. Decision making in this patient demographic should be performed on a case-by-case basis. Long-term clinical evaluation studies and randomized clinical trials are needed for these surgical procedures and their use in the glenohumeral joint to better define surgical indication and efficacy of use, and comparison of efficacy against one another.

DISCLOSURE STATEMENT

The authors have no specific disclosures of or pertaining to the creation of this article. However, disclosures for each authors are as follows: B.M. Saltzman: Nova Science Publishers, Postgraduate Institute for Medicine: Royalties. T. Leroux (no disclosures). B.J. Cole: Aesculap/B.Braun, Cytori, Medipost, National Institutes of Health (National Institute of Arthritis and Musculoskeletal and Skin Diseases and National Institute of Child Health and Human Development): Research support; American Journal of Orthopedics, Arthroscopy, International Cartilage Repair Society, Journal of Bone and Joint Surgery - American, Journal of Shoulder and Elbow Surgery, Journal of the American Academy of Orthopedic Surgeons: Editorial or governing board; American Orthopaedic Society for Sports Medicine, American Shoulder and Elbow Surgeons, Arthroscopy Association of North America: Board or committee member; Arthrex: IP royalties, Paid consultant, Research support; Athletico: Other financial or material support; Carticept: Stock or stock options; DJ Orthopedics, Elsevier Publishing: IP royalties; Össur: Other financial or material support; Regentis: Paid consultant; Stock or stock options; Saunders/Mosby-Elsevier: Publishing royalties, financial or material support; SLACK Incorporated: Publishing royalties, financial or material support; Smith and Nephew: Other financial or material support; Tornier: Other financial or material support; Zimmer: Paid consultant; Research support.

REFERENCES

1. Slabaugh MA, Frank RM, Cole BJ. Resurfacing of isolated articular cartilage defects in the glenohumeral joint with microfracture: a surgical technique & case report. Am J Orthop 2010;39(7):326–32.
2. Patzer T, Lichtenberg S, Kircher J, et al. Influence of SLAP lesions on chondral lesions of the glenohumeral joint. Knee Surg Sports Traumatol Arthrosc 2010; 18:982–7.
3. Provencher MT, Barker JU, Strauss EJ, et al. Glenohumeral arthritis in the young adult. Instr Course Lect 2011;60:137–53.

4. Shin JJ, Mellano C, Cvetanovich GL, et al. Treatment of glenoid chondral defect using micronized allogeneic cartilage matrix implantation. Arthrosc Tech 2014; 3(4):e519–22.

5. Frank RM, Van Thiel GS, Slabaugh MA, et al. Clinical outcomes after microfracture of the glenohumeral joint. Am J Sports Med 2010;38:772–81.

6. Cole BJ, Yanke A, Provencher MT. Nonarthroplasty alternatives for the treatment of glenohumeral arthritis. J Shoulder Elbow Surg 2007;16:231S–40S.

7. Snow M, Funk L. Microfracture of chondral lesions of the glenohumeral joint. Int J Shoulder Surg 2008;2(4):72–6.

8. Romeo AA, Cole BJ, Mazzocca AD, et al. Autologous chondrocyte repair of an articular defect in the humeral head. Arthroscopy 2002;18(8):925–9.

9. Millett PJ, Huffard BH, Horan MP, et al. Outcomes of full-thickness articular cartilage injuries of the shoulder treated with microfracture. Arthroscopy 2009;25(8): 856–63.

10. Steadman JR, Rodkey WG, Rodrigo JJ. Microfracture: surgical technique and rehabilitation to treat chondral defects. Clin Orthop Relat Res 2001;(391 Suppl):S362–9.

11. OUTERBRIDGE GE. The etiology of chondromalacia patellae. J Bone Joint Surg Br 1961;43:742–57.

12. Yeh LR, Kwak S, Kim YS, et al. Evaluation of articular cartilage thickness of the humeral head and glenoid fossa by MR arthrography: anatomic correlation in cadavers. Skeletal Radiol 1998;27(9):500–4.

13. Fox JA, Cole BJ, Romeo AA, et al. Articular cartilage thickness of the humeral head: an anatomic study. Orthopedics 2008;31(3):216.

14. Bicos J, Mazzocca A, Romeo AA. The glenoid center line. Orthopedics 2005; 28(6):581–5.

15. Salata MJ, Kercher JS, Bajaj S, et al. Glenohumeral microfracture. Cartilage 2010; 1(2):121–6.

16. Hsu HC, Luo ZP, Stone JJ, et al. Correlation between rotator cuff tear and glenohumeral degeneration. Acta Orthop Scand 2003;74:89–94.

17. Kang RW, Frank RM, Nho SJ, et al. Complications associated with anterior shoulder instability repair. Arthroscopy 2009;25(8):909–20.

18. Carroll KW, Helms CA, Speer KP. Focal articular cartilage lesions of the superior humeral head: MR imaging findings in seven patients. AJR Am J Roentgenol 2001;176:393–8.

19. Cameron BD, Galatz LM, Ramsey ML, et al. Non-prosthetic management of grade IV osteochondral lesions of the glenohumeral joint. J Shoulder Elbow Surg 2002;11(1):25–32.

20. Fox JA, Cole BJ, Pylawka TK, et al. Chapter 20: cartilage injuries in the shoulder. Stuttgart, Germany: Thieme; 2006.

21. Brown WE, Potter HG, Marx RG, et al. Magnetic resonance imaging appearance of cartilage repair in the knee. Clin Orthop Relat Res 2004;422:214–23.

22. Potter HG, Chong R. Magnetic resonance imaging assessment of chondral lesions and repair. J Bone Joint Surg Am 2009;91(Suppl 1):126–31.

23. Bhatia DN, van Rooyen KS, du Toit DF, et al. Arthroscopic technique of interposition arthroplasty of the glenohumeral joint. Arthroscopy 2006;22:570.e1–5.

24. Van Thiel GS, Riff A, Heard W, et al. Treatment of cartilage defects in young shoulders: from the lab to the clinic. Rush Orthopedics J 2012;3:36–40.

25. Wang VM, Karas V, Lee AS, et al. Assessment of glenoid chondral healing: comparison of microfracture to autologous matrix-induced chondrogenesis in a novel rabbit shoulder model. J Shoulder Elbow Surg 2015;24:1789–800.

26. Gross CE, Chalmers PN, Chahal J, et al. Operative treatment of chondral defects in the glenohumeral joint. Arthroscopy 2012;28(12):1889–901.

27. Kerr BJ, McCarty EC. Outcome of arthroscopic debridement is worse for patients with glenohumeral arthritis of both sides of the joint. Clin Orthop Relat Res 2008; 466(3):634–8.

28. Steadman JR, Rodkey WG, Briggs KK, et al. The microfracture technique in the management of complete cartilage defects in the knee joint. Orthopade 1999; 28(1):26–32.

29. Mithoefer K, Williams RJ 3rd, Warren RF, et al. Chondral resurfacing of articular cartilage defects in the knee with the microfracture technique. Surgical technique. J Bone Joint Surg Am 2006;68(Suppl 1, Pt 2):294–304.

30. Hensley CP, Sum J. Physical therapy intervention for a former power lifter after arthroscopic microfracture procedure for grade IV glenohumeral chondral defects. Int J Sports Phys Ther 2011;6(1):10–26.

31. Siebold R, Lichtenberg S, Habermeyer P. Combination of microfracture and periostal-flap for the treatment of focal full thickness articular cartilage lesions of the shoulder: a prospective study. Knee Surg Sports Traumatol Arthrosc 2003;11:183–9.

32. Buchmann S, Salzmann GM, Glanzmann MC, et al. Early clinical and structural results after autologous chondrocyte transplantation at the glenohumeral joint. J Shoulder Elbow Surg 2012;21:1213–21.

33. Kreuz PC, Steinwachs M, Erggelet C, et al. Classification of graft hypertrophy after autologous chondrocyte implantation of full-thickness chondral defects in the knee. Osteoarthritis Cartilage 2007;15:1339–47.

34. Scheibel M, Barti C, Magosch P, et al. Osteochondral autologous transplantation for the treatment of full-thickness articular cartilage defects of the shoulder. J Bone Joint Surg Br 2004;86(7):991–7.

35. Park TS, Kim TS, Cho JH. Arthroscopic osteochondral autograft transfer in the treatment of an osteochondral defect of the humeral head: report of one case. J Shoulder Elbow Surg 2006;15(6):e31–6.

36. Chapovsky F, Kelly JD IV. Osteochondral allograft transplantation for treatment of glenohumeral instability. Arthroscopy 2005;21(8):1007.e1–4.

37. Saltzman BM, Riboh JC, Cole BJ, et al. Humeral head reconstruction with osteochondral allograft transplantation. Arthroscopy 2015;31(9):1827–34.

38. Kircher J, Patzer T, Magosch P, et al. Osteochondral autologous transplantation for the treatment of full-thickness cartilage defects of the shoulder: results at nine years. J Bone Joint Surg Br 2009;91-B(4):499–503.

39. Beaver RJ, Mahomed M, Backstein D, et al. Fresh osteochondral allografts for post-traumatic defects in the knee. A survivorship analysis. J Bone Joint Surg Br 1992;74:105–10.

40. Zumstein V, Kraljevic M, Hoechel S, et al. The glenohumeral joint–a mismatching system? A morphological analysis of the cartilaginous and osseous curvature of the humeral head and the glenoid cavity. J Orthop Surg Res 2014;9:34–9.

41. Cvetanovich GL, Chalmers PN, Yanke AB, et al. Feasibility of an osteochondral allograft for biologic glenoid resurfacing. J Shoulder Elbow Surg 2014;23:477–84.

42. Chan CM, LeVasseur MR, Lemer AL, et al. Computer modeling analysis of the talar dome as a graft for the humeral head. Arthroscopy 2016;32(8):1671–5.

43. Camp CL, Barlow JD, Krych AJ. Transplantation of a tibial osteochondral allograft to restore a large glenoid osteochondral defect. Orthopedics 2015;38(2): e147–52.

44. Burkhead WZ, Hutton KS. Biologic resurfacing of the glenoid with hemiarthroplasty of the shoulder. J Shoulder Elbow Surg 1995;4:263–70.

45. DePalma AA, Gruson KI. Management of cartilage defects in the shoulder. Curr Rev Musculoskelet Med 2012;5:254–62.

46. Krishnan SG, Burkhead WZ, Nowinski RJ. Humeral hemiarthroplasty with biologic resurfacing of the glenoid and acromion for rotator cuff tear arthropathy. J Tech Shoulder Elbow Surg 2004;5:54–9.

47. Krishnan SG, Nowinski RJ, Harrison D, et al. Humeral hemiarthroplasty with biologic resurfacing of the glenoid for glenohumeral arthritis. J Bone Joint Surg Am 2007;89:727–34.

48. Pennington WT, Bartz BA. Arthroscopic glenoid resurfacing with meniscal allograft: a minimally invasive alternative for treating glenohumeral arthritis. Arthroscopy 2005;21:1517–20.

49. Strauss EJ, Verma NN, Salata MJ, et al. The high failure rate of biologic resurfacing of the glenoid in young patients with glenohumeral arthritis. J Shoulder Elbow Surg 2014;23:409–19.

50. Sweet SJ, Takara T, Ho L, et al. Primary partial humeral head resurfacing: outcomes with the HemiCAP implant. Am J Sports Med 2015;43:579–87.

51. Fortier LA, Hackett CH, Cole BJ. The effects of platelet-rich plasma on cartilage: basic science and clinical application. Oper Tech Sports Med 2011;19:154–9.

52. Smyth NA, Murawski CD, Fortier LA, et al. Platelet-rich plasma in the pathologic process of cartilage: review of basic science evidence. Arthroscopy 2013;29(8): 1399–409.

53. Mascarenhas R, Saltzman BM, Fortier LA, et al. Role of platelet-rich plasma in articular cartilage injury and disease. J Knee Surg 2015;28:3–10.

A Critical Review

Management and Surgical Options for Articular Defects in the Hip

 CrossMark

Eric C. Makhni, MD, MBA[a], Austin V. Stone, MD, PhD[b],
Gift C. Ukwuani, MD[c], William Zuke, BS[c],
Tigran Garabekyan, MD[d], Omer Mei-Dan, MD[e],
Shane J. Nho, MD, MS[c],*

KEYWORDS

- Chondral injury • Osteochondral autologous transplantation
- Osteochondral allograft transplantation • Autologous chondrocyte transplantation
- Mosaicplasty • Viscosupplementation

KEY POINTS

- Nonoperative treatment continues to be the mainstay of treatment for patients with articular cartilage lesions of the hip.
- There is a heterogeneity of support in the scientific literature regarding efficacy of biologic injections for cartilage disease of the hip.
- Treatment algorithms for focal cartilage disease of the hip resemble those for the knee.

INTRODUCTION

Despite significant research and investigative efforts, the optimal management of articular cartilage injury remains a challenge in orthopedic sports medicine **Table 1**. Although much of the research in articular cartilage injuries has occurred in the knee, the recent rapid growth of the hip preservation field, has caused an increase

Disclosures. Nothing to disclose (E.C. Makhni, T. Garabekyan, G.C. Ukwuani, W. Zuke); Smith and Nephew: Research support (A.V. Stone); MITA: Stock or stock Options, Smith & Nephew: Paid consultant; Research support (O. Mei-Dan).

[a] Division of Sports Medicine, Department of Orthopedic Surgery, Henry Ford Health System, 6777 West Maple Road, 3rd Floor East, West Bloomfield, MI 48322, USA; [b] Department of Orthopedic Surgery, Wake Forest School of Medicine, Medical Center Boulevard, Winston-Salem, NC 27157-1070, USA; [c] Division of Hip Preservation Surgery, Rush University Medical Center, 1611 West Harrison Street, Chicago, IL 60612, USA; [d] Southern California Hip Institute, 10640 Riverside Drive, North Hollywood, CA 9160, USA; [e] CU Sports Medicine and Performance Center, University of Colorado, 2150 Stadium Drive, Boulder, CO 80309, USA
* Corresponding author.
E-mail addresses: shane.nho@rushortho.com; nho.research@rushortho.com

Table 1	
Outerbridge classification system for chondromalacia	
Grade	
0	Normal cartilage
1	Softening and swelling of the cartilage
2	Partial-thickness defect with surface fissuring that does not extend to the subchondral bone and is <1.5 cm in diameter
3	Partial-thickness defect with surface fissures extending to the subchondral bone or >1.5 cm in diameter
4	Full-thickness cartilage defect

Data from Outerbridge RE. The etiology of chondromalacia patellae. J Bone Joint Surg Br 1961;43-B:752–7.

in similar emphasis in the hip. The difficulty in treating chondral injury is a direct consequence of the tissue's limited repair capacity. When present in patients undergoing hip arthroscopy for femoroacetabular impingement (FAI) or hip dysplasia, these chondral injuries may be associated with significant pain and decreased patient-reported outcome (PRO) scores when compared with patients without these lesions.[1] Therefore, knowledge of the wide variety of treatment options for these lesions is essential when caring for these patients. Fortunately, many common treatment strategies for articular cartilage lesions in the hip have been adopted from those previously used in the knee, at times with improved success rates due to better joint congruency. These have produced varying degrees of success.[1–4] The goal of this review was to provide an overview of both the nonoperative and operative treatment options for articular cartilage lesions of the hip. The ultimate goal of this treatment is not only to mitigate pain and disability, but also to minimize progression of disease.

CLINICAL PRESENTATION AND DIAGNOSTIC EVALUATION

Patients with articular cartilage lesions of the hip may present with pain and symptoms that may be vague in nature and onset. Often, there may be no discrete event or injury that can be recalled. Therefore, a thorough history and physical examination should be performed for every patient presenting with hip pain and/or disability. Pain is often a chief complaint; therefore, the pain should be described with respect to the nature and location of the pain, exacerbating activities or positions, timing of onset, and position or treatment that provides relief. It is important to identify additional medical comorbidities, patient-specific work or activity-related injuries, or predisposing factors, as these may elucidate concomitant pathologies. Certain sporting activities are known to be associated with chondral injury.[5–9] As with every patient presenting with hip pain or symptoms, other sources of injury must be ruled out, such as lumbo-sacral, urologic, neurologic, or surrounding mimickers that can be perceived as hip pain, such as piriformis syndrome, abductors or adductor tears, and others.

Many patients presenting with FAI have concomitant chondral injury associated with the underlying bony defect. In true pincer-type deformities, the extent of soft tissue injury may be confined to the labrum or be diffuse, causing degeneration, whereas those with CAM deformities are more prone to present with chondral delamination or shear injuries. It is our experience, though, that most patients have a mixed deformity, and as such can suffer from both types of cartilage injuries.

Physical Examination and Imaging Findings

Physical examination is performed in conjunction with thorough history. The examination begins with assessment of patient gait, as we are careful to note existence of any evidence of antalgic gait or abductor lurch. Following gait assessment, laxity evaluation, and standing spinal examination, the patient is positioned supine on the examination table. Any points of tenderness are elicited, such as over the pubic symphysis, groin, ischial tuberosity, or greater trochanter. Both the injured hip, as well as the asymptomatic hip for comparison, are brought through full range of motion arcs in flexion, extension, external rotation, and internal rotation, both in hip flexion and natural hip. Strength is assessed in flexion, extension, and abduction. Finally, provocative maneuvers are then performed. These include impingement testing in the flexion, adduction, and internal rotation position (FADIR). Reproducible pain in this position is often associated with impingement, labral tear, and/or corresponding chondral injury. Dysplastic patients may have a positive test in the setting of labral tear but without impingement. Pain in the FABER position (flexion, abduction, and external rotation) may represent sacro-iliac pathology or posterior impingement if elicited posteriorly but if pain is elicited in the front, this would correspond with inflamed joint or early osteoarthritis. Resisted abduction is performed to elicit any abductor tendinitis or weakness indicative of a tear. Additional tests include lateral rim impingement test, in which pain is elicited with abduction of the hip, indicative of lateral overcoverage, as well as instability tests, which are particularly helpful in patients who have ligamentous laxity or pain following prior hip arthroscopy with possible capsular insufficiency.

Radiographic data may additionally aid in the diagnosis of chondral injury in the hip. Routine imaging includes a plain radiograph series consisting of an anteroposterior pelvis, Dunn lateral, and false profile. Radiographs may be limited in the ability to detect focal chondral disease, and so MRI is routinely used to assess the soft tissue structures. Bony deformity and dysplasia is best visualized with a 3-dimensioinal computed tomography (CT) scan. CT scans also may help demonstrate subchondral cysts that must be identified before surgery. Although the gold standard for diagnosis of chondral lesions remains direct visualization with hip arthroscopy, certain lesions (eg, cysts) require close inspection on preoperative advanced imaging, as these lesions may not be readily evident on "surface" visualization. Direct visualization of the lesion affords accurate measurement of the size, as well as classification, according to any number of cartilage grading systems.

There are several cartilage grading systems available. The Outerbridge classification system is most commonly used and is reproducible and reliable.[10,11] Two less commonly used systems include the Beck classification[12] and the acetabular labrum articular disruption classification.[13]

MANAGEMENT OF PATIENTS WITH CHONDRAL INJURY OF THE HIP
Nonoperative Treatment

Nonoperative treatment remains the mainstay of management for patients with articular cartilage injury of the hip, especially on initial presentation. Initial treatment consists of a trial of rest and/or activity modification, along with anti-inflammatory medications and physical therapy. This treatment protocol may be initiated on clinical diagnosis, along with review of plain radiographs, before obtaining advanced imaging. In our practice, we typically obtain advanced imaging (noncontrast MRI) in patients who fail to respond to treatment after 4 to 6 weeks. When the diagnosis of FAI is confirmed along with possible chondral injury, an intra-articular injection is then offered. This injection is both diagnostic and therapeutic, and response is measured through a postinjection pain diary. Injections are particularly helpful in distinguishing pain sources as being from the hip as opposed to other anatomic sites. A recent systematic review by Lynch and colleagues[14] reported that improved pain relief may be experienced in patients with acetabular chondral injury when compared with those patients with impingement or labral pathology. However, this period of relief may be limited, with recurrence of pain within weeks or months following injection. It is our experience that patients who are older and who may have early degenerative disease, and therefore a large contribution of inflammatory-mediated pain, may experience a longer period of relief than those patients without such findings.

Biologic Injections

A variety of biologic injections exist for treatment of focal and diffuse chondral disease of the hip. These include hyaluronic acid, platelet rich plasma (PRP), and stem cell therapy. Unfortunately, there is still a lack of high-level evidence regarding the efficacy of these treatments in the hip. Moreover, many of the published trials are focused on treatment of hip osteoarthritis, as opposed to focal chondral defects. These studies have demonstrated some benefit to viscosupplementation,[15,16] but these benefits have not been proven in other trials when compared with saline injection.[17,18] Similarly, only limited evidence for PRP exists in this setting. Further studies in patients with focal chondral defects are necessary, however.

SURGICAL OPTIONS FOR CHONDRAL DEFECTS OF THE HIP

As with the knee, it is our preference to use an algorithm-based approach when considering surgery for cartilage defects of the hip (once all nonoperative treatments have failed). Similar to the knee, the first factor to consider is bony "alignment" of the hip joint; namely, the articulation of the acetabular rim with the femoral head/neck junction. Any treatment of cartilage injury from underlying FAI should be addressed intraoperatively, through a removal of the pincer lesion (acetabular rim trimming) and CAM lesion (femoral osteochondroplasty) as evident by preoperative imaging. In cases of significant dysplasia, consideration for a combined arthroscopic and open surgery should be considered for appropriate osteotomy along with the cartilage/labral repair. Second, the stability of the hip should be assessed, especially when considering revision scenarios. It is our experience that many patients with secondary hip instability following initial arthroscopy may experience persistent (or even worse) pain when compared with preoperatively. These symptoms are typically due to lack of a capsular repair during index surgery, or incomplete healing. Therefore, any surgical treatment should consist of capsular repair (or reconstruction if necessary). Finally, the cartilage lesion itself must be addressed, and this can be done according to any of the treatments described as follows.

Articular cartilage defects in the hip may be treated using open[19–25] or arthroscopic techniques.[3,4,6,7,23,26–36] Arthroscopic surgery of the hip continues to grow in popularity for diagnosing and managing articular cartilage injury. Hip arthroscopy demonstrates select advantages for treatment of chondral injury (without significant dysplasia) over open treatment due to improved physical visualization of intra-articular pathology and increased speed of recovery with less soft tissue injury.[28] Open surgery may be warranted as an adjunctive procedure if significant dysplasia or deformity exists. The current arthroscopic techniques for treating hip chondral damage include chondroplasty, microfracture,[4,6,7,26,29,30,32–34,37,38] fibrin adhesives,[35,36] and autologous chondrocyte transplantation (ACT).[27,28,31] Open treatment consists of osteochondral autologous transplantation (OAT) and mosaicplasty,[39] along with osteochondral allograft transplantation.

Chondroplasty

Chondroplasty, or abrasion arthroplasty, is a long-standing debridement technique for partial-thickness chondral lesions that is commonly performed as a component of arthroscopy.[40,41] The primary goal of chondroplasty is to prevent further chondral destabilization, pain, and mechanical symptoms by resultant chondral flaps. These injuries typically occur as a result of shearing at the chondrolabral junction, often producing a "wave" sign and later a true cartilage flap. This represents a delamination of the cartilage from the underlying subchondral bone. It is our practice to attempt to keep the cartilage grossly intact despite this delamination, when possible, as opposed to unroofing and debriding the defect. Once debrided, there often remains an area of full-thickness, Grade IV cartilage injury that requires further treatment, and often microfracture (see the next section). Alternatively, when concomitant labral pathology exists, it is our preference to try to incorporate the cartilage delamination into the repair construct (**Fig. 1**), with the goal of eventual stabilization and healing. Additionally, anchor placement adjacent to the articular cartilage delamination is thought to induce bleeding behind the cartilage and stimulate a healing response.

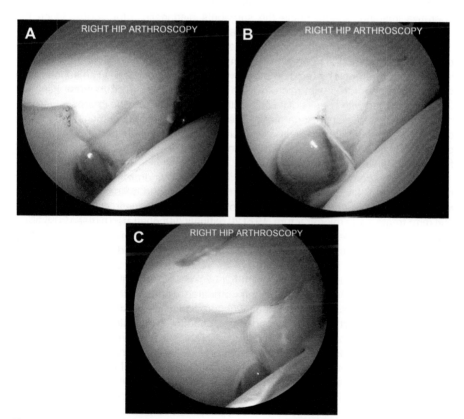

Fig. 1. Incorporation of cartilage delamination (*A*) into labral repair construct (*B, C*), left hip. Note the prominent "wave sign" indicating cartilage delamination from the underlying FAI. (*Courtesy of* Dr Shane J. Nho, Chicago, IL.)

Microfracture

Microfracture is a widely used technique in the knee that has seen widespread use for the management of chondral defects in the hip.[1,4,6,7,26,29,30,32–34,37,38,42–45] The indications for microfracture in the reported techniques follow those described in the knee,[44,45] and are rapidly evolving in their use in the femoral head and acetabulum.[4,32,38,46] Classically, in the knee, microfracture is indicated in for full-thickness chondral lesions measuring less than 2 cm^2 with corresponding good to excellent clinical results.[44,45] In our practice, microfracture in the hip is a first-line treatment for full-thickness cartilage defects provided there is a stable rim of cartilage surrounding the defect.

The same values have been recommended in the hip for focal, full-thickness defect of less than 2 cm^2 and minimal radiographic arthritis (Tönnis grade 0–1)[8,26,29,30,32–34,47]; however, a recent case series has suggested full-thickness defects of up to 7.50 cm^2 may be effectively managed with microfracture.[4] The investigators further advocate that hip arthroscopy may be used in older patients with Tönnis grade 0 or 1 despite good to excellent results in 60% at 2-year follow-up.[4] Patients with Tönnis grade 2 changes demonstrate increased conversion to total hip arthroplasty at 2 years following hip arthroscopy; consequently Tönnis grade 2 is considered a relative exclusion criteria.[48]

Microfracture can be performed during hip arthroscopy in the standard supine position, as previously described.[38] The patient history and physical, combined with preoperative imaging, should guide the surgeon's diagnostic arthroscopy. Once the chondral lesion is identified, unstable cartilage should be removed from the subchondral bone (**Fig. 2**). A ring curette may then be used to create a perpendicular edge from the defect's subchondral bone to the healthy cartilage to contain the marrow clot during microfracture, thereby removing the layer of calcified cartilage. The subchondral bone is then perforated with microfracture awls. Acetabular microfracture also may be accomplished with the use of flexible drills,[46] which may provide improved perpendicular access to lesions. Regardless of technique, a bleeding response should be confirmed from the subchondral bone to ensure adequate penetration.[32,46] Depth of penetration should be 4 mm with perforations spaced at least 2 to 3 mm apart to avoid fracture of the subchondral plate.

Reported outcomes demonstrate that microfracture is an effective technique for managing full-thickness chondral defects. Karthikeyan and colleagues[30] found that in their 20-patient series with a mean age of 37 years and a mean chondral defect of 154 mm^2 treated with microfracture, 19 of 20 patients demonstrated a mean 96% filling of the microfracture defect at second-look arthroscopy. Philippon and colleagues[34] reported similar defect fillings of 95% to 100% at the time of second-look arthroscopy in their 9-patient series with a mean age of 37 years and mean acetabular defect of 1.63 cm^2. Microfracture for patients with full-thickness chondral defects continue to do well at 3 years postoperatively when compared with a matched cohort that did not undergo microfracture.[43] A 35-patient cohort with a full-thickness chondral defect that underwent hip arthroscopic chondral microfracture was matched to a 70-patient cohort that did not undergo microfracture.[43] No statistical differences were found in PROs between the groups. A recent systematic review by MacDonald and colleagues[32] examined microfracture as an adjunct treatment for chondral defects in FAI and identified positive outcomes in 266 of 267 patients. The complication rate was 0.7%, and 1.1% required revision surgery. Microfracture may be effective (see **Fig. 2**) even in large lesions (>2 cm^2) and in older patients (>50 years) rather than limited to more conventional lesion sizes (<2 cm^2).[4] Continued exploration of the techniques and outcomes for microfracture may result in expanded indications for microfracture treatment.

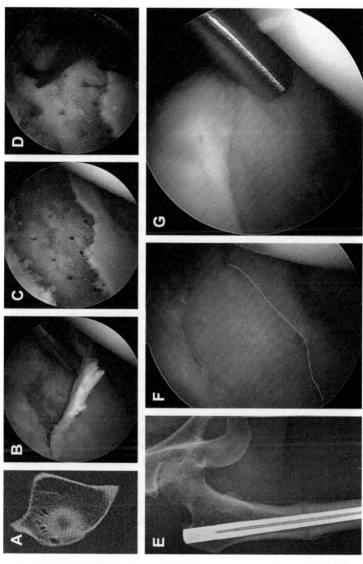

Fig. 2. Microfracture of large acetabular chondral defect. Right hip with evidence of cystic and cartilage disease (*A*) due to femoral retro-torsion and CAM type FAI with corresponding arthroscopic appearance (*B*) undergoing labral reconstruction. After debridement of the unstable cartilage flap, the defect was microfractured using a drill (Stryker, Phoenix, AZ) (*C*), with evidence of bleeding subchondral bone indicating adequate microfracture (*D*). A derotational osteotomy was then performed to correct (−15) degrees of femoral torsion to normal values (*E*). Corresponding images with second-look arthroscopy, demonstrating well-incorporated reconstructed labrum (tensor fascia lata [TFL] allograft) with excellent fill of the defect (*F, G*) in setting of prior procedure. (*Courtesy of* Dr Omer Mei-Dan, Boulder, CO.)

Autologous Chondrocyte Transplantation

ACT is an evolving treatment strategy for cartilage repair. ACT is a 2-stage operation that extracts viable chondrocytes, cultures them in a laboratory setting, and finally reimplants the chondrocytes in a second surgical procedure. Reimplantation techniques vary, but like microfracture techniques, ACT for the hip has been adopted from the knee literature.[49–52] An alternative to ACT is autologous matrix-induced chondrogenesis (AMIC), which is a single-stage procedure to attempt recreation of hyaline cartilage.[53] The indications for performing ACT and AMIC are classically a larger chondral defect (3 cm^2 or larger) with a focal, full-thickness Outerbridge grade 3 or 4 defect and minimal radiographic evidence of osteoarthritis (Tönnis 1 or less).[1,27,28,31] In comparison with the microfracture literature, a systematic review recently identified that lesions in the hip treated with arthroscopic ACT were significantly larger than those treated with microfracture.[1] As the techniques and technologies continue to advance, the indications may be expanded for autologous chondrocyte transplantation and chondrogenesis techniques.

Arthroscopic technique for ACT in the hip may be performed after routine hip arthroscopy and in conjunction with additional procedures. Fontana and colleagues[28] described taking an initial cartilage sample at the time of diagnostic arthroscopy. Following a 30-day incubation period, the patient returns for a second operation in which the chondral lesion is prepared with debridement and a chondrocyte culture on bioresorbable 3-dimensional scaffolding is prepared for implantation. The graft is cut precisely to fit the defect and introduced arthroscopically.[28] Alternative scaffolds also have been described and the implantation techniques are similar.[27,31] The AMIC technique, which is similar to ACT, is described as a single-stage operation.[53] In AMIC, the chondral defect is again arthroscopically debrided in a standard fashion but microfracture is then performed. After microfracture of the defect, a bioresorbable scaffolding is placed over the microfracture defect.[53]

Outcomes for ACT and AMIC are promising. In a case-control comparison between ACT and AMIC, the modified Harris Hip Score (mHHS) was statistically improved at 5-year follow-up in both groups but the improvement was not statistically different between groups.[53] The mean defect size was 2.8 ± 0.7 cm^2 in the ACT group (n = 26) and 2.9 ± 0.8 cm^2 in the AMIC group (n = 31).[53] Subgroup analysis demonstrated successful improvement in both groups for defect sizes greater than 3 cm^2, and the investigators concluded that AMIC could be effectively applied to larger defects.[53] Fickert and colleagues[27] reported that 3-dimensional ACT could be effective for larger defects (mean 3.5 cm^2) at 1-year follow-up as measured by significant and maintained improvements in the Nonarthritic Hip Score (NHS), mHHS, and Short Form (SF)-36 scores. A smaller case series (n = 6) reported on arthroscopic 3-dimensional ACT reported similar improvement to Fickert and colleagues[27] as measured by NHS and WOMAC scores. With further development of AMIC, ACT may become less desirable due to its staged requirement; however, both techniques demonstrate optimistic early results.

Cartilage Repair

Fibrin adhesive is a proposed option for arthroscopic repair of chondral delamination.[35,36] The initial results are promising; however, the patient series are small. Stafford and colleagues[35] treated 43 hips with chondral delamination by microfracturing under the flap and securing the flap with fibrin glue. At 28 months of follow-up, the pain and function mHHS subscales remained improved. Tzaveas and Villar[36] treated delaminated cartilage injury arthroscopically with fibrin glue. At 1-year follow-up, the mHHS overall and pain scores remained improved. Sekiya and colleagues[54] reported a single case in which a 1-cm^2 chondral flap was secured with suture after microfracture. The mHHS and Hip Outcome Score (HOS)–Activities of Daily Living and HOS–Sport-Specific Subscales were improved at 2 years.[54] A recent biomechanical study in cadavers examining arthroscopic chondral repair techniques identified early biomechanical failure in fibrin adhesive repair, which failed after only 50 cycles.[55] The same study evaluated suture repair of chondral flaps and found that it was stable throughout the 1500-cycle testing regimen.[55] The small number of reported outcomes and early laboratory failure may limit fibrin's clinical use; however, both fibrin glue and suture repair warrant further investigation.

Bone Grafting and Osteochondral Grafting for Osteochondral Defects of the Hip

Many of the previously described techniques are well-suited for chondral disease that spares the subchondral plate; however, when large (>0.5 cm^2) full-thickness osteochondral defects are present, treatment should be directed at bone-grafting procedure. Traditionally, osteochondral autograft or allograft transplantation offer an alternative to ACT and AMIC for larger osteochondral defects. This approach is described in the following paragraphs. However, one of the senior authors (O.M.-D.) from this group has described a technique for bone grafting of large osteochondral defects that may be performed as a primary procedure. Although this technique does not provide cartilage transplantation, it does serve as an initial procedure that may obviate the need for an open dislocation of the hip and good bone fill, enabling a good base for cartilage growth.[56]

In this procedure,[56] the lesion is identified and debrided completely, exposing the overlying subchondral bone. A microfracture awl (XL Microfracture awl; Smith and Nephew, Andover, MA) is used to penetrate and probe the defect, thus exposing the underlying cyst and bone defect. A drill (Micro FX; Stryker, Phoenix, AZ) is used to incite bleeding and eventual healing from the base of the cyst. A curved shaver (4.5-mm curved shaver 30° Double Bite; Stryker, Kalamazoo, MI) is then used with the central blade portion removed and subsequent packing of bone graft (DBZ; Synthes, Westchester, PA) into the outer barrel. The removed inner blade is then used to impact the graft into the defect with precision. This technique may be used in the acetabular side (as described in the referenced technique article[56]), or in the femoral head, as seen in **Fig. 3**.

Unlike microfracture, ACT, and AMIC, osteochondral grafting requires surgical dislocation of the hip. The indications have been adopted from the knee literature[22,42,57–60] and include larger osteochondral defects in patients with Tönnis grade 0 or 1 disease. Mosaicplasty is similar to OAT, but combines multiple plugs for larger defects. This treatment strategy has been applied to multiple diseases and trauma due to its ability to manage larger defects.[1,19,20]

The technique for OAT and mosaicplasty is adopted from the knee. Meyers[60] reported using fresh osteochondral allograft in hips with osteonecrosis. The cylindrical allograft was selected and press-fit to match the articular contour of the femoral head similar to the technique used for the knee.[60] Krych and colleagues[22] used a comparable OAT technique for acetabular defects. Mosaicplasty is usually performed with autologous osteochondral grafts and multiple cylindrical plugs are combined to fill larger lesions. Emre and colleagues[19] describe the use of osteochondral autograft to treat an osteochondral lesion in the femoral head through a standard Smith-Peterson approach and surgical dislocation. Autologous plugs may be taken from the ipsilateral knee through a mini-open approach.[19]

Outcomes for OAT and mosaicplasty demonstrate improvement, but are associated with greater morbidity in comparison with the arthroscopic techniques as a

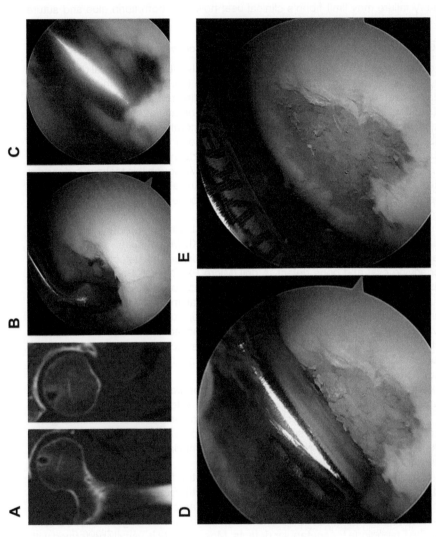

Fig. 3. Bone grafting of a femoral head cyst using a curved shaver. Large cystic lesion noted in the femoral head on preoperative CT images (*A*) with intraoperative debridement and curettage pictures (*B*). Bone grafting delivered through curved shaver using technique referenced and described by senior author (OMD) (*C, D*). Final appearance of cystic lesion with bone grafting (*E*). (*Courtesy of* Dr Omer Mei-Dan, Boulder, CO.)

result of the surgical dislocation and autologous donor site. A case report by Evans and Providence[61] reported success in a femoral head fresh OAT with full painless range of motion at 1-year follow-up, although the report was limited to 1 patient. The 2 patients with OAT for acetabular lesions reported by Krych and colleagues[22] remained improved at 2-year and 3-year follow-ups with respective mHHS scores of 97 and 100.

Mosaicplasty outcomes in the hip are also limited and primarily confined to case reports and small case series. Nam and colleagues[24] and Hart and colleagues[21] reported on a total of 3 patients treated with mosaicplasty and saw return to activities without pain. In 1 series of 10 patients with large femoral head lesions by Girard and colleagues,[62] at more than 2 years postoperatively, the mean HHS was maintained at 80, increased from 53 preoperatively. OAT and mosaicplasty are technically demanding and have increased morbidity in the hip compared with the knee, which have limited their use and their outcomes reporting. These treatments may remain an effective strategy for treating large osteochondral lesions in the femoral head and acetabulum in patients without radiographic evidence of osteoarthritis.

SUMMARY

The management of articular cartilage defects in the hip remains a challenging but very important area of rapidly evolving treatment strategies. As the understanding of cartilage biology continues to grow, nonoperative and operative techniques will likely involve a greater biologic focus. Arthroscopic techniques continue to decrease morbidity and offer innovative solutions and new applications for microfracture, ACT, and AMIC. This may be especially true with cystic conditions of the acetabulum or femoral head that may benefit from bone grafting arthroscopically, as referenced and illustrated in this article. The indications for cartilage-preserving techniques continue to expand and new biologics offer innovative solutions that may provide benefit to the patient.

REFERENCES

1. Marquez-Lara A, Mannava S, Howse EA, et al. Arthroscopic management of hip chondral defects: a systematic review of the literature. Arthroscopy 2016;32(7): 1435–43.
2. Bedi A, Feeley BT, Williams RJ 3rd. Management of articular cartilage defects of the knee. J Bone Joint Surg Am 2010;92(4):994–1009.
3. Lubowitz JH. Editorial commentary: microfracture for focal cartilage defects: is the hip like the knee? Arthroscopy 2016;32(1):201–2.
4. Trask DJ, Keene JS. Analysis of the current indications for microfracture of chondral lesions in the hip joint. Am J Sports Med 2016;44(12):3070–6.
5. Guanche CA, Sikka RS. Acetabular labral tears with underlying chondromalacia: a possible association with high-level running. Arthroscopy 2005;21(5):580–5.
6. McDonald JE, Herzog MM, Philippon MJ. Return to play after hip arthroscopy with microfracture in elite athletes. Arthroscopy 2013;29(2):330–5.
7. McDonald JE, Herzog MM, Philippon MJ. Performance outcomes in professional hockey players following arthroscopic treatment of FAI and microfracture of the hip. Knee Surg Sports Traumatol Arthrosc 2014;22(4):915–9.
8. Singh PJ, O'Donnell JM. The outcome of hip arthroscopy in Australian football league players: a review of 27 hips. Arthroscopy 2010;26(6):743–9.

9. Stone AV, Howse EA, Mannava S, et al. Cyclists have greater chondromalacia index than age-matched controls at the time of hip arthroscopy. Arthroscopy 2016; 32(10):2102–9.

10. Cameron ML, Briggs KK, Steadman JR. Reproducibility and reliability of the Outerbridge classification for grading chondral lesions of the knee arthroscopically. Am J Sports Med 2003;31(1):83–6.

11. Outerbridge RE. The etiology of chondromalacia patellae. J Bone Joint Surg Br 1961;43-B:752–7.

12. Beck M, Leunig M, Parvizi J, et al. Anterior femoroacetabular impingement: part II. Midterm results of surgical treatment. Clin Orthop Relat Res 2004;(418):67–73.

13. Callaghan JJ, Robenberg AG, Rubash HE. The adult hip. 2nd edition. Philadelphia: Lippincott Williams & Wilkins; 2007.

14. Lynch TS, Steinhaus ME, Popkin CA, et al. Outcomes after diagnostic hip injection. Arthroscopy 2016;32(8):1702–11.

15. Migliore A, Granata M, Tormenta S, et al. Hip viscosupplementation under ultrasound guidance reduces NSAID consumption in symptomatic hip osteoarthritis patients in a long follow-up. Data from Italian registry. Eur Rev Med Pharmacol Sci 2011;15(1):25–34.

16. Migliore A, Massafra U, Bizzi E, et al. Intra-articular injection of hyaluronic acid (MW 1,500-2,000 kDa; HyalOne) in symptomatic osteoarthritis of the hip: a prospective cohort study. Arch Orthop Trauma Surg 2011;131(12):1677–85.

17. Atchia I, Kane D, Reed MR, et al. Efficacy of a single ultrasound-guided injection for the treatment of hip osteoarthritis. Ann Rheum Dis 2011;70(1):110–6.

18. Qvistgaard E, Christensen R, Torp-Pedersen S, et al. Intra-articular treatment of hip osteoarthritis: a randomized trial of hyaluronic acid, corticosteroid, and isotonic saline. Osteoarthr Cartil 2006;14(2):163–70.

19. Emre TY, Cift H, Seyhan B, et al. Mosaicplasty for the treatment of the osteochondral lesion in the femoral head. Bull NYU Hosp Jt Dis 2012;70(4):288–90.

20. Gagala J, Tarczynska M, Gaweda K. Clinical and radiological outcomes of treatment of avascular necrosis of the femoral head using autologous osteochondral transfer (mosaicplasty): preliminary report. Int Orthop 2013;37(7):1239–44.

21. Hart R, Janecek M, Visna P, et al. Mosaicplasty for the treatment of femoral head defect after incorrect resorbable screw insertion. Arthroscopy 2003;19(10):E1–5.

22. Krych AJ, Lorich DG, Kelly BT. Treatment of focal osteochondral defects of the acetabulum with osteochondral allograft transplantation. Orthopedics 2011; 34(7):e307–11.

23. Logan ZS, Redmond JM, Spelsberg SC, et al. Chondral lesions of the hip. Clin Sports Med 2016;35(3):361–72.

24. Nam D, Shindle MK, Buly RL, et al. Traumatic osteochondral injury of the femoral head treated by mosaicplasty: a report of two cases. Hss j 2010;6(2):228–34.

25. Sotereanos NG, DeMeo PJ, Hughes TB, et al. Autogenous osteochondral transfer in the femoral head after osteonecrosis. Orthopedics 2008;31(2):177.

26. Domb BG, Redmond JM, Dunne KF, et al. A matched-pair controlled study of microfracture of the hip with average 2-year follow-up: do full-thickness chondral defects portend an inferior prognosis in hip arthroscopy? Arthroscopy 2015; 31(4):628–34.

27. Fickert S, Schattenberg T, Niks M, et al. Feasibility of arthroscopic 3-dimensional, purely autologous chondrocyte transplantation for chondral defects of the hip: a case series. Arch Orthop Trauma Surg 2014;134(7):971–8.

28. Fontana A, Bistolfi A, Crova M, et al. Arthroscopic treatment of hip chondral defects: autologous chondrocyte transplantation versus simple debridement–a pilot study. Arthroscopy 2012;28(3):322–9.

29. Haviv B, Singh PJ, Takla A, et al. Arthroscopic femoral osteochondroplasty for cam lesions with isolated acetabular chondral damage. J Bone Joint Surg Br 2010;92(5):629–33.

30. Karthikeyan S, Roberts S, Griffin D. Microfracture for acetabular chondral defects in patients with femoroacetabular impingement: results at second-look arthroscopic surgery. Am J Sports Med 2012;40(12):2725–30.

31. Korsmeier K, Classen T, Kamminga M, et al. Arthroscopic three-dimensional autologous chondrocyte transplantation using spheroids for the treatment of full-thickness cartilage defects of the hip joint. Knee Surg Sports Traumatol Arthrosc 2016;24(6):2032–7.

32. MacDonald AE, Bedi A, Horner NS, et al. Indications and outcomes for microfracture as an adjunct to hip arthroscopy for treatment of chondral defects in patients with femoroacetabular impingement: a systematic review. Arthroscopy 2016; 32(1):190–200.e2.

33. Philippon MJ, Briggs KK, Yen YM, et al. Outcomes following hip arthroscopy for femoroacetabular impingement with associated chondrolabral dysfunction: minimum two-year follow-up. J Bone Joint Surg Br 2009;91(1):16–23.

34. Philippon MJ, Schenker ML, Briggs KK, et al. Can microfracture produce repair tissue in acetabular chondral defects? Arthroscopy 2008;24(1):46–50.

35. Stafford GH, Bunn JR, Villar RN. Arthroscopic repair of delaminated acetabular articular cartilage using fibrin adhesive. Results at one to three years. Hip Int 2011;21(6):744–50.

36. Tzaveas AP, Villar RN. Arthroscopic repair of acetabular chondral delamination with fibrin adhesive. Hip Int 2010;20(1):115–9.

37. Domb BG, Gupta A, Dunne KF, et al. Microfracture in the hip: results of a matched-cohort controlled study with 2-year follow-up. Am J Sports Med 2015; 43(8):1865–74.

38. McGill KC, Bush-Joseph CA, Nho SJ. Hip microfracture: indications, technique, and outcomes. Cartilage 2010;1(2):127–36.

39. Cetinkaya S, Toker B, Taser O. Arthroscopic retrograde osteochondral autologous transplantation to chondral lesion in femoral head. Orthopedics 2014; 37(6):e600–4.

40. Sansone V, de Girolamo L, Pascale W, et al. Long-term results of abrasion arthroplasty for full-thickness cartilage lesions of the medial femoral condyle. Arthroscopy 2015;31(3):396–403.

41. Yen YM, Kocher MS. Chondral lesions of the hip: microfracture and chondroplasty. Sports Med Arthrosc 2010;18(2):83–9.

42. El Bitar YF, Lindner D, Jackson TJ, et al. Joint-preserving surgical options for management of chondral injuries of the hip. J Am Acad Orthop Surg 2014; 22(1):46–56.

43. Lodhia P, Gui C, Chandrasekaran S, et al. Microfracture in the hip: a matched-control study with average 3-year follow-up. J Hip Preservation Surg 2015;2(4):417–27.

44. Steadman JR, Briggs KK, Rodrigo JJ, et al. Outcomes of microfracture for traumatic chondral defects of the knee: average 11-year follow-up. Arthroscopy 2003;19(5):477–84.

45. Steadman JR, Miller BS, Karas SG, et al. The microfracture technique in the treatment of full-thickness chondral lesions of the knee in National Football League players. J Knee Surg 2003;16(2):83–6.

46. Haughom BD, Erickson BJ, Rybalko D, et al. Arthroscopic acetabular microfracture with the use of flexible drills: a technique guide. Arthrosc Tech 2014;3(4): e459–63.
47. Byrd JW, Jones KS. Arthroscopic femoroplasty in the management of cam-type femoroacetabular impingement. Clin Orthop Relat Res 2009;467(3):739–46.
48. Chandrasekaran S, Darwish N, Gui C, et al. Outcomes of hip arthroscopy in patients with Tönnis grade-2 osteoarthritis at a mean 2-year follow-up. Evaluation using a matched-pair analysis with Tönnis grade-0 and grade-1 cohorts. J Bone Joint Surg Am 2016;98(12):973–82.
49. Bartlett W, Skinner JA, Gooding CR, et al. Autologous chondrocyte implantation versus matrix-induced autologous chondrocyte implantation for osteochondral defects of the knee: a prospective, randomised study. J Bone Joint Surg Br 2005;87(5):640–5.
50. Biant LC, Bentley G, Vijayan S, et al. Long-term results of autologous chondrocyte implantation in the knee for chronic chondral and osteochondral defects. Am J Sports Med 2014;42(9):2178–83.
51. Gooding CR, Bartlett W, Bentley G, et al. A prospective, randomised study comparing two techniques of autologous chondrocyte implantation for osteochondral defects in the knee: periosteum covered versus type I/III collagen covered. Knee 2006;13(3):203–10.
52. Knutsen G, Drogset JO, Engebretsen L, et al. A randomized trial comparing autologous chondrocyte implantation with microfracture. Findings at five years. J Bone Joint Surg Am 2007;89(10):2105–12.
53. Mancini D, Fontana A. Five-year results of arthroscopic techniques for the treatment of acetabular chondral lesions in femoroacetabular impingement. Int Orthop 2014;38(10):2057–64.
54. Sekiya JK, Martin RL, Lesniak BP. Arthroscopic repair of delaminated acetabular articular cartilage in femoroacetabular impingement. Orthopedics 2009;32(9).
55. Cassar-Gheiti AJ, Byrne DP, Kavanagh E, et al. Comparison of four chondral repair techniques in the hip joint: a biomechanical study using a physiological human cadaveric model. Osteoarthr Cartil 2015;23(6):1018–25.
56. Garabekyan TC, Chadayammuri V, Pascual-Garrido C, et al. Arthroscopic bone grafting of deep acetabular cysts using a curved delivery device. Arhtroscopy Tech 2016;5(1):113–9.
57. Alford JW, Cole BJ. Cartilage restoration, part 2: techniques, outcomes, and future directions. Am J Sports Med 2005;33(3):443–60.
58. Beaver RJ, Mahomed M, Backstein D, et al. Fresh osteochondral allografts for post-traumatic defects in the knee. A survivorship analysis. J Bone Joint Surg Br 1992;74(1):105–10.
59. Emmerson BC, Gortz S, Jamali AA, et al. Fresh osteochondral allografting in the treatment of osteochondritis dissecans of the femoral condyle. Am J Sports Med 2007;35(6):907–14.
60. Meyers MH. Resurfacing of the femoral head with fresh osteochondral allografts. Long-term results. Clin Orthop Relat Res 1985;(197):111–4.
61. Evans KN, Providence BC. Case report: fresh-stored osteochondral allograft for treatment of osteochondritis dissecans the femoral head. Clin Orthop Relat Res 2010;468(2):613–8.
62. Girard J, Roumazeille T, Sakr M, et al. Osteochondral mosaicplasty of the femoral head. Hip Int 2011;21(5):542–8.

The Early Osteoarthritic Knee

Implications for Cartilage Repair

Chaitu Malempati, DO, Cale A. Jacobs, PhD, ATC,
Christian Lattermann, MD*

KEYWORDS

- Knee • Articular cartilage • Osteoarthritis • Cartilage defect • Bone marrow lesion
- Extracellular matrix • Body mass index

KEY POINTS

- Patients with early knee osteoarthritis (OA) are more likely to have inferior long-term outcomes or earlier graft failure.
- Cartilage repair procedures are more likely to fail in the early OA knee due to a chronic synovial and chondrogenic process, which is confounded by persistent muscle weakness and altered pain processing for those with increased preoperative symptom duration.
- Pain, radiographic changes, patient-reported outcomes (PROs), and macroscopic changes on arthroscopic evaluation or MRI can assist clinicians in identifying the early OA knee to both aid in clinical decision making and create realistic postoperative expectations for patients.

INTRODUCTION

Patients with early OA have been reported to have inferior outcomes with an increased prevalence of early failure after cartilage procedures.[1] Both after osteochondral allograft and after cell-based (autologous chondrocyte implantation [ACI]) procedures, the worst performing groups with regard to survival of the original graft are patients with early OA.[1,2] The underlying reasons for this failure are unknown and likely multifactorial in nature. The purpose of this review is to identify (1) the underlying factors associated with poorer results following cartilage repair for this subset of patients and (2) methods to better identify patients with early OA, which often is difficult in the clinical setting.

Dr C. Lattermann is supported by the NIH-NIAMS K-23 award (5K23AR060275).
Department of Orthopaedic Surgery and Sports Medicine, University of Kentucky, Kentucky Clinic K416, 740 South Limestone, Lexington, KY 40536, USA
* Corresponding author.
E-mail address: clatt2@uky.edu

WHY ARE PATIENTS WITH EARLY OSTEOARTHRITIS MORE LIKELY TO FAIL CARTILAGE PROCEDURES?

It is no secret that patients with early OA have worse outcome scores overall and are expected to fail earlier. The underlying reasons for failure in this group have not been established; however, the etiology is likely multifactorial and includes the duration of symptoms, muscular weakness, and chronic synovial and chondrogenic inflammation.

Duration of Symptoms

Accepting that chronic inflammation is a feature of early OA, it is clinically relevant to record the earliest onset of symptoms. In particular, joint swelling is the clinical correlate to significant joint inflammation. Several reports in recent years have pointed out the importance of duration of clinical symptoms, such as recurrent effusions and pain prior to chondral repair.[3,4] Symptoms exhibited for more than 1 year are associated with overall worse patient-related outcomes after chondral repair regardless if a cell-based technique or a chondral plug transfer is performed, and this finding has been demonstrated by both adolescent and adult patients.[3,5,6]

There are multiple factors as to why the duration of preoperative symptoms may negatively influence postoperative outcome, and the factors are likely not mutually exclusive. First, as is discussed, longer duration of symptoms is likely associated with the joint being in a state of synovial and chondrogenic inflammatory state for a longer period of time. As such, longer duration of symptoms has been associated with worse arthroscopic International Cartilage Repair Society (ICRS) grades, which are indicative of more extensive chondral changes.[7] Second, the longer that pain is present during the preoperative period, the more likely central nervous system adaptations are to occur.[8] As such, prolonged symptom duration prior to surgical intervention may promote the creation of a cycle of chronic pain that coincides with progressive chondral changes. Patients respond to OA-related pain differently, and different pain phenotypes have been identified.[9,10] Some patients demonstrate characteristics of pain centralization, including lower pain thresholds and self-reports of severe pain despite mild radiographic changes whereas some patients' response in exactly the opposite manner with low pain sensitivity and more efficient descending inhibition despite the presence of progressive radiographic changes.[9,10] Patients with altered pain processing may then be at greater risk of persistent postoperative pain, and future studies are necessary to determine if adjunctive pain neuroscience education or other psychological or behavioral science interventions can improve postoperative outcomes for this at-risk subset of patients.[11]

Muscular Weakness

Additionally, presence of severe preoperative muscular atrophy and deconditioning has been reported to persist postoperatively.[12–16] Both eccentric and concentric quadriceps strength before chondral repair procedures are reduced by a 20% to 30% compared with the opposite leg.[12–16] Unfortunately, after chondral repair procedures, this weakness is amplified over the course of the first postoperative year.[13] Patients undergoing tibiofemoral ACI procedures drop to 50% of their preoperative strength at 6 months after surgery and only regain their preoperative eccentric and concentric quadriceps strength at 1 year after surgery.[13] Furthermore, Loken and colleagues[15] reported marked strength deficits at mean 7 years after ACI. This is of significant concern for the progression of OA because the protective muscular envelope dysfunction is unable to reduce contact load in these individuals. This severe lack of strength recovery may partially be influenced by recurrent effusions and inflammation but may also be a consequence of chronic changes in the ultrastructure of the quadriceps musculature.[17]

Synovial and Chondrogenic Inflammation

Recently it has been learned that synovial inflammation may be an important factor for the initiation and progress of early OA. Angele and colleagues[18] evaluated more than 400 patients undergoing an autologous cell scaffold–based chondrocyte transplantation technique, showing that the level of interleukin (IL)-1 gene expression and conversely the reduction of collagen type II (CTX-II) gene expression in the autologous chondrocytes prior to reimplantation was predictive of surgical failure at less than 2 years. That suggests that inflammatory cytokines in conjunction with signs of chondrodestruction (both features of early OA) clearly affect the outcome of these procedures. In this study the investigators focused on the innate production of inflammatory cytokines within the harvested chondrocytes, indicating that chondrocytes may already display an activated chronic inflammatory phenotype.[18]

The author has recently been able to show that even in the very early stages after ACL injury (an injury known to predispose a joint for early OA) patterns of chronic inflammation surface within a few days after injury up to 4 weeks after injury.[19,20] In particular, the proinflammatory cytokine IL-1 is expressed early on and increases over the first 4 weeks after injury accompanied by a drop in the anti-inflammatory cytokine IL-1ra.[20] Consequently a significant rise in collagen breakdown has been demonstrated characterized through a 250% increase of the C-telopeptide of CTX-II.[20] Although the author was not able to link this pattern of inflammation to success of failure of a chondral procedure, the CTX-II level at the time of surgery was predictive of worse clinical outcome at 2 years after injury and explained 37% (model: CTX-II alone; $r^2 = 0.32$) of the variation of KOOS quality-of-life scores. In women, it even explained 52% (model: CTX-II + female gender; $r^2 = 0.52$) of the variation.[21] These data suggest that a more sensitive measure than radiograph is clearly needed to define the stage of OA to better predict success and failure of chondral repair.

HOW CAN THE EARLY OSTEOARTHRITIS KNEE BE IDENTIFIED IN THE CLINICAL SETTING?

The methods to clinically identify the early OA knee were first established by Luyten and colleagues[22] and were recently adapted by Madry and colleagues.[23] In short, this system defines the early OA knee as a patient (1) with frequent, persistent pain; (2) without radiographic evidence of moderate or severe joint space narrowing; and (3) with macroscopic articular cartilage changes present either by arthroscopic evaluation or MRI (**Fig. 1**).[23]

Pain

Early OA classification criteria[22,23]: at least 2 episodes of pain in the past year, each lasting 10 days or more.

Pain is the primary criteria for the classification of early OA, or better termed, symptomatic early OA. As previously discussed, pain and radiographic severity are not synonymous in that there are subsets of OA patients with severe pain with mild radiographic changes and those with mild or no pain despite severe radiographic changes.[9,10] In addition, treatment of cartilage lesions in the absence of pain has yielded inferior clinical results.[24,25] As such, the goal is not to simply identify those with imaging results consistent with OA but rather to identify the symptomatic early OA patient to better identify the optimal treatment plan.

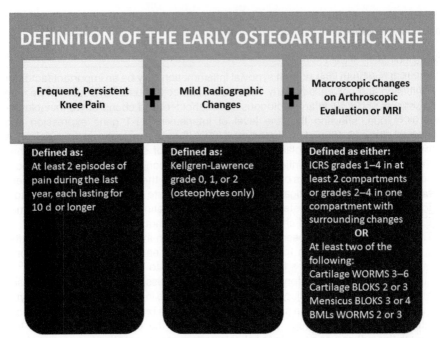

Fig. 1. Three criteria necessary to classify the early OA knee. (*Adapted from* Luyten FP, Denti M, Filardo G, et al. Definition and classification of early osteoarthritis of the knee. Knee Surg Sports Traumatol Arthrosc 2011;20:401–6; and Madry H, Kon E, Condello V, et al. Early osteoarthritis of the knee. Knee Surg Sports Traumatol Arthrosc 2016;24(6):1753–62.)

Building on the pain criteria set forth by Luyten and colleagues,[22] collecting detailed information about the specific nature of the patient's pain, may also return useful clinical information. First, it is important to note the different mechanisms and processing characteristics of movement-elicited pain and pain at rest in the knee OA patient, because the two are not significantly correlated with one another.[26] Movement-elicited pain is more related to the local tissue response and is directly related to peripheral nociceptor stimulation. Pain at rest, however, is the result of both peripheral input and central processing.[27] Chronic peripheral nociceptor stimulation can cause hyperexcitability of the central nervous system, resulting in increasing pain intensity and/or duration that are disproportionate to the true peripheral input, or simply put, the patient reports pain that is worse than their radiographs.[9,26–28]

This central adaptation becomes more likely the longer that pain is present — a process that is embodied by the progressive knee OA process. Movement-elicited pain, specifically, pain when navigating stairs, has been identified as the first activity to denote the progression of OA.[29] In a study of more than 4600 patients, Hensor and colleagues[29] reported that the first activity to become symptomatic was navigating stairs, followed in order by walking and standing. Then, after affecting progressing from more physically demanding tasks like stairs to less-demanding tasks like standing over time, central processing alterations seem to take root as patients then begin to report pain at rest, including when lying, sitting, or in bed.[29]

When considering surgical treatment options for early OA patients, it is important to record not only the frequency and duration of pain as suggested by Luyten and colleagues[22] and Madry and colleagues[23] but also whether the patient is experiencing pain at rest in addition to movement-elicited pain because it may have implications on the patients postoperative recovery. Although not specifically evaluated in cartilage repair patients, Lundblad and colleagues[26] reported that preoperative pain at rest was indicative of pain at rest 18 months after total knee arthroplasty. As such, patients who report pain at rest or pain that is disproportionate to clinical and imaging evaluation results, or those with other risk factors for persistent postoperative pain, such as depression or anxiety, may require adjunctive interventions to ensure a successful surgical treatment. Identifying and referring at-risk patients preoperatively has been demonstrated to improve outcomes after spine surgery,[30,31] and future studies are necessary to determine if similar practices can also improve outcomes after knee cartilage procedures for this subset of patients.

Radiographic Assessment

Early OA classification criteria[22,23]: Kellgren-Lawrence grade 0, 1, or 2 (only osteophytes).

In the Kellgren-Lawrence definition, the early OA patient is identified as one who does not have evidence of joint space narrowing but could have mild osteophyte formation per the Kellgren-Lawrence grading scale.[32] The Multicenter Anterior Cruciate Ligament Revision Study consortium evaluated several routinely used radiographic grading scales for the assessment of OA.[33] Although the International Knee Documentation Committee (IKDC) classification demonstrated slightly better reliability than the Kellgren-Lawrence and other scales, the Kellgren-Lawrence classification better correlated with arthroscopic findings. Specifically, both the correlation with arthroscopic findings and inter-rater reliability were improved when based on Rosenberg radiographs. As such, it is recommended that the posteroanterior weight-bearing radiograph with the knee flexed to 45° be used when determining the radiographic OA grade.[33]

Arthroscopic Evaluation

Early OA classification criteria[22,23]: ICRS grades 1 to 4 in at least 2 compartments or ICRS grades 2 to 4 in 1 compartment with surrounding softening and swelling.

The arthroscopic evaluation remains the gold standard for assessing cartilage defects and their reparability. The location, grade, size, depth, and morphology or character of a cartilage defect can be assessed with relative ease as well as whether the lesion is monofocal, bifocal, or multifocal. Any suspicious, smooth surfaces can be probed to assess the integrity of the articular cartilage. Furthermore, when assessing a cartilage defect, any fissures and tissue surrounding the defect should be carefully palpated with a probe to determine the integrity of the surrounding cartilage. The anteroposterior, medial-lateral, and depth measurements can then be recorded and the degree of containment of the lesion can also be assessed, all of which may later aid in clinical decision making and/or operative planning. Although the arthroscopic evaluation is an invaluable tool in the assessment of cartilage defects in addition to ligamentous stability, meniscal appearance, and arthritic changes, the arthroscopic evaluation cannot determine the cause of the lesion, and should, of course, be accompanied by a thorough history and clinical examination.

The ICRS arthroscopic classification system focuses on the depth of the lesion and the area of damage.[34] ICRS grades range from 0 (normal) to 4 (severely abnormal) based on the features of the lesion.[34] When used in the identification of the early OA knee, the ICRS classification is simplified to include knees with lesions of any severity in 2 compartments, or, for those with only 1 compartment affected, lesions that extend down greater than 50% of the depth of the cartilage with surrounding soft-ening and swelling that may be indicative of more diffuse OA changes.[22,23]

MRI

Early OA classification criteria (at least 2)[22,23]: cartilage morphology, Whole-Organ Magnetic Resonance Imaging Score (WORMS) 3 to 6, cartilage Boston Leeds Osteo-arthritis Knee Score (BLOKS) grade 2 or 3, meniscus BLOKS grade 3 or 4, and bone marrow lesions (BMLs) WORMS 2 or 3.

Although the WORMS score was developed to generate a grade or score to esti-mate the sum total of the changes to the joint as a whole, only 1 specific evaluation was included in the identification of the early OA knee.[22,23] Using fat-suppressed, T2-weighted, fast spin-echo images, the early OA knee was defined as having a min-imum of multiple areas of partial-thickness loss with areas of normal thickness or a focal lesion with diameter greater than 1 cm but less than 75% of the bony region.[35] In addition, a feature of early OA was defined as BMLs affecting 25% or more of any bony region (anterior, middle, or posterior third of the medial or lateral femoral con-dyles or of the medial or lateral tibial plateau).[22,23,35]

Similarly, the BLOKS was developed to sum the osteoarthritic changes for the knee as a whole but only 2 specific features of this detailed scoring system have been used to define the early OA knee.[22] The minimum requirement in the definition of early OA is a cartilage BLOKS grade of 2, which is associated with cartilage loss of between 10% and 75% of an individual compartment.[36] In addition, displaced meniscal tears or par-tial resection and more severe tearing, maceration, or resection are considered indic-ative of early OA.[36]

The combination of these MRI findings has been associated with the presence of early OA; however, both the chronicity of the BML and the combined presence of BML with local articular cartilage defects must be considered. It has been well estab-lished that chronic BMLs associated with degenerative cartilage lesions are a tell-tale sign of progressive OA, and OA patients with BMLs more frequently require total knee arthroplasty than those without BMLs.[37,38] Furthermore, Felson and colleagues[39] reported that knee pain is correlated with either the development of BML or enlarge-ment of any preexisting lesions. In the OA knee, these lesions do not resolve but prog-ress in concert with chondral degeneration. If the articular cartilage is interrupted, it can no longer shield the underlying bone from cyclic mechanical and hydrodynamic stress. As a result, the combination of mechanical forces and fluid shift through the lesion site create a persistent cycle of bone remodeling and pain.[39–41] Unfortu-nately, with respect to chondral repair, these readily identifiable lesions are features of advanced-stage OA and, when present, preclude chondral repair procedures.

On the contrary, acute BMLs as well as those with no local articular cartilage changes may resolve. Acute BMLs are most commonly seen after acute knee injuries, such as ACL injuries. They occur in close to 100% of patients and are associated with the development of significant chondral lesions over time.[42,43] Lattermann and col-leagues[42] analyzed the data form a subcohort of the Multicenter Orthopaedic Out-comes Network (MOON) and were able to show that the presence, volume, or distribution of bone bruises at the time of injury alone are no predictor of clinical symp-toms consistent with the onset of early OA. Unlike the traditional OA knee, a majority of acute BMLs are not associated with local articular cartilage changes. As such, the articular cartilage can shield the subchondral bone from increased forces and prevent cyclic fluid shift within the BML, thus allowing the cycle of chronic bone remodeling to be broken. Although acute BMLs seem to resolve regardless of initial size[42,44]; it must not be forgotten that BMLs with identifiable chondral lesions at the time of surgery predict worse outcome and a clinically symptoms associated with early OA as early as 6 years after ACL reconstruction.[42]

Using Patient-Reported Outcomes to Identify At-Risk Patients

Although not specifically addressed in the definition of the early OA knee,[22,23] PRO scores may also be used to identify both the early OA knee and patients who more likely to demonstrate inferior outcomes after cartilage procedures. Englund and colleagues[45] previously established a PRO-based definition of symptomatic early OA based on patients' responses to the Knee and Osteoarthritis Outcome Score (KOOS). Per their definition, a knee was considered to demonstrate symptoms consistent with early OA radiographic based on the following criteria:

1. At least 50% of the responses to the questions used to calculate the KOOS Knee-related Quality of Life (KRQOL) subscale were less than the best possible response and the KOOS KRQOL subcomponent score was less than or equal to 87.5.
2. Similar criteria were met for at least 2 of the remaining 4 KOOS subscales (at least 50% of each subscale responses were less than the best possible response with subcomponent scores below the following thresholds: pain less than or equal to 86.1, symptoms less than or equal to 85.7, activities of daily living less than or equal to 86.8, sports and recreation less than or equal to 85.0).[45]

In addition to identifying the early OA knee, the Lysholm and IKDC scores can be used to identify patients who may have inferior postoperative outcomes. Howard and Lattermann[46] reported that patients who have Lysholm scores greater than 41 and IKDC scores greater than 35 are more than 7 times more likely to demonstrate meaningful postoperative changes in PROs after ACI. This then means that patients with scores below these thresholds are at much greater risk of having a poor outcome after a cartilage procedure. This information can then be used to identify an early OA knee and/or at-risk patients to aid in clinical decision making as well as to create realistic postoperative expectations when counseling patients prior to surgery.

SUMMARY

Patients with early OA have been reported to have inferior outcomes with an increased prevalence of early failure after cartilage procedures.[1,2] As such, it is imperative that the early OA knee be identified both to better inform clinical decisions and to also create more realistic postoperative expectations for the patient. Pain, radiographic changes, PROs, and macroscopic changes on arthroscopic evaluation or MRI can assist clinicians in the identification of the early OA knee.[22,23,45,46] In addition, future studies are necessary to determine if chronic pain-related adjunctive interventions may improve postoperative outcomes for patients at the greatest risk of a poor outcome due to maladaptive pain processing.

REFERENCES

1. Minas T, Von Keudell A, Bryant T, et al. A minimum 10-year outcome study of autologous chondrocyte implantation. Clin Orthop Relat Res 2014;472:41–51.
2. Briggs DT, Sadr KN, Pulido PA, et al. The use of osteochondral allograft transplantation for primary treatment of cartilage lesions in the knee. Cartilage 2015; 6(4):203–7.
3. Harris JD, Siston RA, Pan X, et al. Autologous chondrocyte implantation: a systematic review. J Bone Joint Surg Am 2010;92(12):2220–33.

4. Ollat D, Lebel B, Thaunat M, et al. Mosaic osteochondral transplantations in the knee joint, midterm results of the SFA multicenter study. Orthop Traumatol Surg Res 2011;97(8 Suppl):S160–6.

5. DiBartola AC, Wright BM, Magnussen RA, et al. Clinical outcomes after autologous chondrocyte implantation in adolescents' knees: a systematic review. Arthroscopy 2016;32(9):1905–16.

6. Ebert JR, Smith A, Edwards PK, et al. Factors predictive of outcome 5 years after matrix-induced autologous chondrocyte implantation in the tibiofemoral joint. Am J Sports Med 2013;41(6):1245–54.

7. Cuellar VG, Cuellar JM, Kirsch T, et al. Correlation of synovial fluid biomarkers with cartilage pathology and associated outcomes in knee arthroscopy. Arthroscopy 2016;32(3):475–85.

8. Latremoliere A, Woolf CJ. Central sensitization: a generator of pain hypersensitivity by central neural plasticity. J Pain 2009;10:895–926.

9. Finan PH, Buenaver LF, Bounds SC, et al. Discordance between pain and radiographic severity in knee osteoarthritis: findings from quantitative sensor testing of central sensitization. Arthritis Rheum 2013;65(2):363–72.

10. Egsgaard LL, Eskehave TN, Bay-Jensen AC, et al. Identifying specific profiles in patients with different degrees of painful knee osteoarthritis based on serological biochemical and mechanistic pain biomarkers: a diagnostic approach based on cluster analysis. Pain 2015;156(1):96–107.

11. Louw A, Zimney K, Puentedura EJ, et al. The efficacy of pain neuroscience education on musculoskeletal pain: a sysetmatic review of the literature. Physiother Theory Pract 2016;32(5):332–55.

12. Thoma LM, Flanigan DC, Chaudhari AM, et al. Quadriceps femoris strength and sagittal-plane knee biomechanics during stair descent in individuals with articular cartilage defects in the knee. J Sport Rehabil 2014;23(3):259–69.

13. Howard JS, Mattacola CG, Mullineaux DR, et al. Patient-oriented and performance-based outcomes after knee autologous chondrocyte implantation: a timeline for the first year of recovery. J Sport Rehabil 2014;23(3):223–34.

14. Muller S, Hirschmuller A, Erggelet C, et al. Significantly worse isokinetic hamstring-quadriceps ratio in patellofemoral compared to condylar defects 4 years after autologous chondrocyte implantation. Knee Surg Sports Traumatol Arthrosc 2015;23(8):2151–8.

15. Loken S, Ludvigsen TC, Hoysveen T, et al. Autologous chondrocyte implantation to repair knee cartilage injury: ultrastructural evaluation at 2 years and long-term follow-up including muscle strength measurements. Knee Surg Sports Traumatol Arthrosc 2009;17(11):1278–88.

16. Schmitt LC, Quatman CE, Paterno MV, et al. Functional outcomes after surgical management of articular cartilage lesions in the knee: A sysetmatic literature review to guide postoperative rehabilitation. J Orthop Sports Phys Ther 2014;44(8): 565–78.

17. Noehren B, Andersen A, Hardy P, et al. Cellular and morphological alterations in the vastus lateralis muscle as the result of ACL injury and reconstruction. J Bone Joint Surg Am 2016;98(18):1541–7.

18. Angele P, Fritz J, Albrecht D, et al. Defect type, localization and marker gene expression determines early adverse events of matrix-associated autologous chondrocyte implantation. Injury 2015;46(Suppl 4):S2–9.

19. Lattermann C, Jacobs CA, Proffitt Bunnell M, et al. A multicenter study of early anti-inflammatory treatment in patients with acute ACL tear. Am J Sports Med 2016;45(2):325–33.

20. Lattermann C, Jacobs CA, Proffitt Bunnell M, et al. Logistical challenges and design considerations for studies using acute anterior cruciate ligament injury as a potential model for early posttraumatic arthritis. J Orthop Res 2016. [Epub ahead of print].

21. Lattermann C, Jacobs CA, Whale Conley C, et al. Biomarkers on the day of ACL reconstruction and sex predictive of knee-related quality of life at 2-year follow-up. AOSSM Specialty Day. San Diego, CA, March 18, 2017.

22. Luyten FP, Denti M, Filardo G, et al. Definition and classification of early osteoarthritis of the knee. Knee Surg Sports Traumatol Arthrosc 2011;20:401–6.

23. Madry H, Kon E, Condello V, et al. Early osteoarthritis of the knee. Knee Surg Sports Traumatol Arthrosc 2016;24(6):1753–62.

24. Widuchowski W, Widuchowski J, Koczy B, et al. Untreated asymptomatic deep cartilage lesions associated with anterior cruciate ligament injury: results at 10- and 15-year follow-up. Am J Sports Med 2009;37:688–92.

25. Mithoefer K, Saris DBF, Farr J, et al. Guidelines for the design and conduct of clinical studies in knee articular cartilage repair: International Cartilage Repair Society recommendations based on current scientific evidence and standards of clinical care. Cartilage 2011;2(2):100–21.

26. Lundblad H, Kreicbergs A, Jansson KA. Prediction of persistent pain after total knee replacement for osteoarthritis. J Bone Joint Surg Br 2008;90-B:166–71.

27. Malfait A-M, Schnitzer TJ. Towards a mechanism-based approach to pain management in osteoarthritis. Nat Rev Rheumatol 2013;9:654–64.

28. Grosu I, Lavand'homme P, Thienpont E. Pain after knee arthroplasty: an unresolved issue. Knee Surg Sports Traumatol Arthrosc 2014;22:1744–58.

29. Hensor EMA, Dube B, Kingsbury SR, et al. Toward a clinical definition of early osteoarthritis: onset of patient-reported knee pain begins on the stairs. Data from the Osteoarthtitis Initiative. Arthritis Care Res 2015;67(1):40–7.

30. Elsamadicy AA, Adogwa O, Cheng J, et al. Pretreatment of depression before cervical spine surgery improves patients' perception of postoperative health status: a retrospective, single institution experience. World Neurosurg 2016;87: 214–9.

31. Adogwa O, Elsamadicy AA, Cheng J, et al. Pretreatment of anxiety before cervical spine surgery improves clinical outcomes: a prospective, single-institution experience. World Neurosurg 2016;88:625–30.

32. Kellgren JH, Lawrence JS. Radiological assessment of osteoarthritis. Ann Rheum Dis 1957;16:494–502.

33. Wright RW, Group TM. Osteoarthritis classification scales: interobserver reliability and arthroscopic correlation. J Bone Joint Surg Am 2014;96(14):1145–51.

34. Brittberg M, Aglietti P, Gambardella R, et al. The ICRS clinical cartilage injury evaluation system. 2000. Available at: http://cartilage.org/content/uploads/2014/10/ICRS_evaluation.pdf. Accessed December 13, 2016.

35. Peterfy CG, Guermazi A, Zaim S, et al. Whole-organ magnetic resonance imaging score (WORMS) of the knee in osteoarthritis. Osteoarthritis Cartilage 2004;12: 177–90.

36. Hunter DJ, Lo GH, Gale D, et al. The reliablity of a new scoring system for knee osteoarthritis MRI and the validity of bone marrow lesion assessment: BLOKS (Boston Leeds Osteoarthritis Knee Score). Ann Rheum Dis 2008;67(2):206–11.

37. Scher C, Craig J, Nelson F. Bone marrow edema in the knee in osteoarthritis and association with total knee arthroplasty within a three-year period. Skeletal Radiol 2008;37:609–17.

38. Dore D, Quinn S, Ding S, et al. Natural history and clinical significance of MRI-detected bone marrow lesions at the knee: a prospective study in community dwelling older adults. Arthritis Res Ther 2010;12:R223.
39. Felson DT, Niu J, Guermazi A, et al. Correlation of the development of knee pain with enlarging bone marrow lesions on magnetic resonance imaging. Arthritis Rheum 2007;56(9):2986–92.
40. Sharkey PF, Cohen SB, Leinberry CF, et al. Subchondral bone marrow lesions associated with knee osteoarthritis. Am J Orthop 2012;41(9):413–7.
41. Hwang J, Bae WC, Shieu W, et al. Increased hydraulic conductance of human articular cartilage and subchondral bone plate with progression of osteoarthritis. Arthritis Rheum 2008;58(12):3831–42.
42. Lattermann C, Jacobs CA, Reinke EK, et al. Are bone bruise characteristics and articular cartilage pathology associated with inferior outcomes two and six years after anterior cruciate ligament reconstruction? Cartilage, in press.
43. Potter HG, Jain SK, Ma Y, et al. Cartilage injury after acute, isolated anterior cruciate ligament tear: immediate and longitudinal effect with clinical/MRI follow-up. Am J Sports Med 2012;40:276–85.
44. Costa-Paz M, Muscolo DL, Ayerza M, et al. Magnetic resonance imaging follow-up sudy of bone bruises associated with anterior cruciate ligament ruptures. Arthroscopy 2001;17(5):445–9.
45. Englund M, Roos EM, Lohmander LS. Impact of type of meniscal tear on radiographic and symptomatic knee osteoarthritis. a sixteen-year followup of menisectomy with matched controls. Arthritis Rheum 2003;48(8):2178–87.
46. Howard JS, Lattermann C. Use of preoperative patient reported outcome scores to predict outcome following autologous chondrocyte implantation. Orthop J Sports Med 2014;2(Suppl 2).

Index

Note: Page numbers of article titles are in **boldface** type.

A

Acetaminophen, in articular cartilage disease, 450
Allografts, **509–523**
    osteochondral, 437, 438, 439, 440, 446
        background of, 510
        cryopreserved viable (shell allograft), 515–516
        future directions in, 516–517
        in articular defects of shoulder, 566–567
        indications for, 517
        infection associated with, 518–519
        outcomes of, 512–515, 516, 518
        rehabilitation following, 517–518
        screening, procurement, and storage of, 511–512
        surgical considerations in, 516
        technical considerations in, 512, 513, 514, 517
        uses of, 510
    particulated articular cartilage for, 516–517
Ankle, osteochondritis dissecans of, nonsurgical treatment of, 481
        patient evaluation in, 480–481
        surgical treatment of, 481–482
Articular cartilage, basic science of, **413–425**
    chondrocytes of, 416, 417–418
        in vitro and chondrogenic strategy choice, 419–420
    collagen in, 415
    function of, 415
    inflammatory mediators of, 416–419
    injury of, arthrography in diagnosis of, 429, 431, 432
        MRI imaging in, 428
    mature, extracellular matrix of, 415–416
    of distal femur, 413–414
    particulated, for allografts, 516–517
    proteoglycans of, 416
    response to injury, 420–421
    synovial cartilage and, 415
Articular cartilage disease, bracing in, 449
    exercise and, 448
    nonoperative options for, **447–456**
    oral medications in, 449–450
    physical therapy/strength training in, 449
    prolotherapy (and biologics) in, 453–454
    steroid injections in, 452
    supplements in, 451–452

Clin Sports Med 36 (2017) 597–601
http://dx.doi.org/10.1016/S0278-5919(17)30044-3
0278-5919/17

Printed and bound by CPI Group (UK) Ltd, Croydon, CR0 4YY

08/05/2025

01864701-0004

Moving?

Make sure your subscription moves with you!

To notify us of your new address, find your **Clinics Account Number** (located on your mailing label above your name), and contact customer service at:

Email: journalscustomerservice-usa@elsevier.com

800-654-2452 (subscribers in the U.S. & Canada)
314-447-8871 (subscribers outside of the U.S. & Canada)

Fax number: 314-447-8029

Elsevier Health Sciences Division
Subscription Customer Service
3251 Riverport Lane
Maryland Heights, MO 63043

*To ensure uninterrupted delivery of your subscription, please notify us at least 4 weeks in advance of move.